GERMAN MEDICAL DATA SCIENCES 2022 – FUTURE MEDICINE: MORE PRECISE, MORE INTEGRATIVE, MORE SUSTAINABLE!

Studies in Health Technology and Informatics

International health informatics is driven by developments in biomedical technologies and medical informatics research that are advancing in parallel and form one integrated world of information and communication media and result in massive amounts of health data. These components include genomics and precision medicine, machine learning, translational informatics, intelligent systems for clinicians and patients, mobile health applications, data-driven telecommunication and rehabilitative technology, sensors, intelligent home technology, EHR and patient-controlled data, and Internet of Things.

Studies in Health Technology and Informatics (HTI) series was started in 1990 in collaboration with EU programmes that preceded the Horizon 2020 to promote biomedical and health informatics research. It has developed into a highly visible global platform for the dissemination of original research in this field, containing more than 250 volumes of high-quality works from all over the world.

The international Editorial Board selects publications with relevance and quality for the field. All contributions to the volumes in the series are peer reviewed.

Volumes in the HTI series are submitted for indexing by MEDLINE/PubMed; Web of Science: Conference Proceedings Citation Index – Science (CPCI-S) and Book Citation Index – Science (BKCI-S); Google Scholar; Scopus; EMCare.

Volume 296

Recently published in this series

ISSN 0926-9630 (print)
ISSN 1879-8365 (online)

German Medical Data Sciences 2022 – Future Medicine: More Precise, More Integrative, More Sustainable!

Proceedings of the Joint Conference of the 67th Annual Meeting of the German Association of Medical Informatics, Biometry, and Epidemiology e.V. (gmds) and the 14th Annual Meeting of the TMF – Technology, Methods, and Infrastructure for Networked Medical Research e.V. 2022 online in Kiel, Germany

Edited by

Rainer Röhrig
Editor-in-Chief
Institute of Medical Informatics, University Hospital RWTH Aachen, Germany

Niels Grabe
GMDS – Technical Committee Medical Bioinformatics and Systems Biology
Tissue Imaging & Analysis Center, Heidelberg University, Germany

Verena S. Hoffmann
GMDS – Technical Committee Biometrics
Institute of Medical Informatics, Biometrics and Epidemiology, Ludwig-Maximilian University, Munich, Germany

Ursula Hübner
GMDS – Technical Committee Medical Informatics
Health Informatics Research Group, Osnabrück University of Applied Sciences, Germany

Jochem König
GMDS – Technical Committee Epidemiology
Institute of Medical Biostatistics, Epidemiology and Informatics, University Medicine Mainz, Germany

Ulrich Sax
GMDS – Technical Committee Medical Informatics
Department Medical Bioinformatics, University Medicine Göttingen, Germany

Björn Schreiweis
Chair of the joint Scientific Programm Committee of GMDS and TMF
Institute for Medical Informatics and Statistics, Kiel University and University Hospital Schleswig-Holstein, Kiel, Germany

Martin Sedlmayr
GMDS – Congress Secretary
Institute for Medical Informatics, Technische Universität Dresden, Germany

IOS Press

Amsterdam • Berlin • Washington, DC

ISBN 978-1-64368-302-7 (print)
ISBN 978-1-64368-303-4 (online)
Library of Congress Control Number: 2022943325
doi: 10.3233/SHTI296

Cover image by Björn Schreiweis, Kiel

Publisher
IOS Press BV
Nieuwe Hemweg 6B
1013 BG Amsterdam
Netherlands
fax: +31 20 687 0019
e-mail: order@iospress.nl

For book sales in the USA and Canada:
IOS Press, Inc.
6751 Tepper Drive
Clifton, VA 20124
USA
Tel.: +1 703 830 6300
Fax: +1 703 830 2300
sales@iospress.com

Future Medicine:
More Precise, More Integrative,
More Sustainable!

Foreword by Michael Krawczak and Björn Bergh
Congress Presidents

The aim of medical research is to gain scientific knowledge which will serve to improve the diagnosis, therapy and prevention of diseases. In the course of this, it is also becoming increasingly important to account for the changing framework conditions of medical care. We live in an aging society. This not only leads to greater use of medical care, but also puts the human resources and infrastructural basis of the health system under great pressure. Elderly people need more frequent and more complex medical help, which makes the widespread lack of nursing and medical staff ever more obvious, especially in rural areas.

The effects of this development cannot be countered by economic and political measures alone. Rather, the current demographic, sociological and technical changes call for science-based solutions which can better adapt medical action to the needs of patients. This is not just about the development of more precisely tailored drugs, or of biomarkers for the improved early detection of disease. New and advanced technical and methodological developments are also of particular importance in medical research. These developments will allow better access, networking and research use of data, information and knowledge. All of this is required to facilitate progress in research and care with the aim of ensuring that medicine remains affordable and accessible for everybody in the future. The examples of important developments are many: in addition to applications of artificial intelligence which allow researchers to analyze increasingly complex clinical and molecular data, and which have already begun to make their way into healthcare practice in many places, this includes innovative methods for the self-collection of health data by patients.

Under the motto "Medicine in Transition – More Precise, More Integrative, More Sustainable", the German Society for Medical Informatics, Biometry and Epidemiology (GMDS) and the Technology and Methods Platform for Networked Medical Research (TMF) have organized a conference from 21–25 August 2022 which addresses the challenges and opportunities of digitization in the healthcare sector. This event has been long in the planning, and it had been hoped that it would take place in Kiel, the capital of Schleswig-Holstein. It was a new edition of the conference previously planned for 2021 in Kiel which ultimately had to be held online due to the corona pandemic. Unfortunately, the 2022 event has met with the same fate because the so-called "summer wave" of the pandemic has once again caused a massive increase in the number of infections nationwide. Those responsible for the meeting therefore hope all the more that a face-to-face professional exchange on current topics in medical informatics, biometrics, epidemiology and medical documentation will finally be possible again in 2023.

The corona pandemic has not only disrupted the planning of many events, it has also impressively demonstrated the importance of technical and methodological aspects of digitization for the functionality of a modern healthcare system. Even if the nature and the extent of the lessons learned still leave a lot to be desired, the problems of the past always represent an opportunity for the future. From the point of view of the organizers, the forthcoming 2022 joint conference of TMF and GMDS offers an ideal platform to work out these opportunities in professional discourse and deliver the impetus to then use them in our daily practice.

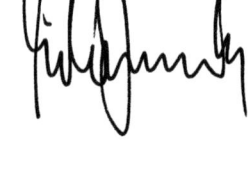

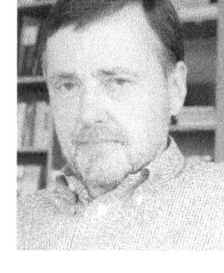

Prof. Dr. Michael Krawczak
Congress president TMF

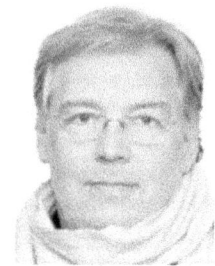

Prof. Dr. Björn Bergh
Congress President GMDS

The Future of the Data Sciences — Integrative and Sustainable

Foreword by Harald Binder
President of GMDS

It is a pleasure to offer some thoughts on the occasion of this volume of contributions as part of the 67th Annual Meeting of the German Association for Medical Informatics, Biometry and Epidemiology (GMDS) organized jointly with the 13th Annual Congress of the German TMF (Technology, Methods, and Infrastructure for Networked Medical Research).

The conference motto points to the need for an integrative approach in medicine to facilitate change and achieve sustainability. The medical data sciences represented by the GMDS and TMF are an integral part of the medical landscape, so our call for integration and sustainability is also targeted at ourselves. Indeed, the integration of the – sometimes quite heterogeneous – landscape of data sciences is not only a nice-to-have feature, but is key to advancing biomedical research and healthcare with our contributions. This can be a tough challenge at times, not least due to entrenched ways of doing things within disciplines, but it is not only possible but also enjoyable to come together across disciplines. The GMDS provides a platform for such a coming together of disciplines, and we strive to do this not only nationally, but also to connect to the internationally emerging medical data-science community. One of the prime outcomes can be seen in this volume, and I hope that you will enjoy reading it, maybe even more when viewed through an integrative lens.

Yours sincerely,

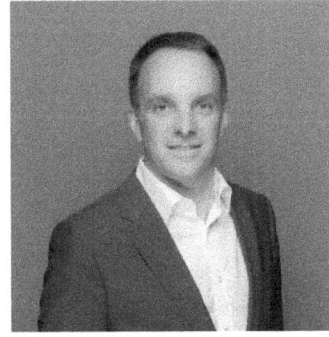

Prof. Dr. Harald Binder
President of the GMDS

German Medical Data Sciences 2022
Preface for the 6th Volume

Preface by the Editorial Board and the Scientific Program Committee

At the time of the submission of contribution, we assumed that we would be able to hold the joint meeting of TMF and GMDS as a live event. Despite this prospect, the number of paper submissions has decreased, especially the number of full papers (Table 1). One possible reason for the decrease in submissions may be the proximity of the deadline to the MIE2022 deadline (EFMI-conference Medical Informatics Europe 2022, Nice)[1] and the deadline for the submission of applications in the Medical Informatics Initiative.

Table 1. Contributions submitted by subject and type of submission 2022, compared with 2021. There may have been other abstract submissions (poster and talk) that are not included in these statistics. (see text)

Subject	GMS MIBE	Stud HTI	Talk	Poster	Sum 2022	Sum 2021	2022 vs 2021
Medical Informatics	1	27	37	26	**91**	112	-19%
Biometry			16	1	**17**	25	-32%
Epidemiology			12	4	**16**	17	-6%
Bioinformatics and System Biology		1	3		**4**	8	-50%
Clinical and epidemiological studies			5		**5**	4	25%
Interdisipliary		3	16	7	**26**	19	37%
Public Health	1	1	9	3	**14**	15	-7%
Sum 2022	**2**	**32**	**98**	**41**	**173**	206	-16%
Sum 2021	7	52	101	44			
2022 vs. 2021	-71%	-38%	-3%	-7%			

Acceptance rates were 100% among the full papers submitted, (1 of 1) for contributions to GMS MIBE and 44% (14 of 32)[2] for contributions to Studies in Health Technology and Informatics (Stud HTI). One contribution to the MIBE was withdrawn during the review process, and one contribution to Stud HTI was withdrawn after final acceptance. The complete review process is shown in Fig. 1. Due to technical constraints, the figure (and statistics) do not include the withdrawn abstracts.

We wish you an exciting conference and an inspiring reading of the proceedings.

(Editor in Chief GMDS in Stud HTI) Rainer Röhrig
(Bioinformatics and Systems Medicine) Tim Beißbarth
(Biometrics) Verena Hoffmann
(Medical Informatics) Ursula Hübner
(Bioinformatics and Systems Medicine) Nils Grabe
(Editor in Chief GMS MIBE) Petra Knaup-Gregori
(Epidemiology) Jochem König
(Medical Informatics) Ulrich Sax
(Chair of SPC) Björn Schreiweis
(Congress Secretary) Martin Sedlmayr

---

[1] 65 full papers was submitted from Germany for MIE 2022, Nice
[2] For comparison, acceptance rate of full paper at MIE 2022, 54% (147 of 271).

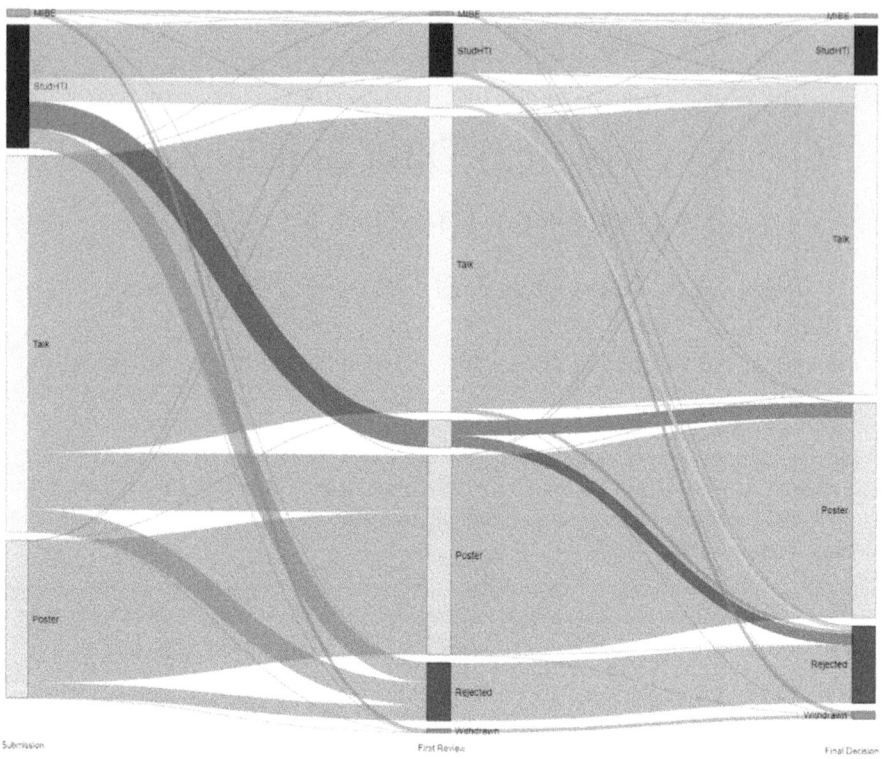

Figure 1. The submitted contributions (left) and the prelimanary and final decision on acceptance after the peer review process (right). Blue = full paper. Yellow = Abstracts, Red = Rejected in peer review or withdrawn by authors after peer review process startet. (Withdrawal of abstracts was not fully recorded.)

Reviewers for GMDS & TMF 2022

The members of the Editorial Board and the Scientific Program Committee would like to thank all reviewers for the joint annual meeting of GMDS and TMF 2022

Klutke, Peter
Knaup-Gregori, Petra
Kock-Schoppenhauer, Ann-Kristin
Kombeiz, Alexander
Konietschke, Frank
Kossen, Robert
Kraft, Bodo
Kraska, Detlef
Kraus, Stefan
Krefting, Dagmar
Kremer, Lisanne
Krumkamp, Ralf
Kusch, Harald
Kutafina, Ekaterina
Lablans, Martin
Lehmann, Christoph
Leverkus, Friedhelm
Liedtke, Wenke
Lipprandt, Myriam
Löbe, Matthias
Lux, Thomas
Majeed, Raphael W.
Marschollek, Michael
Mejia, Luisa
Moorthy, Preetha
Müller-Mielitz, Stefan
Naumann, Laura
Nehmiz, Gerhard
Niekrenz, Lukas
Niemeyer, Anna
Nyoungui, Elisabeth Félicité
Otto, Ronny
Otto-Sobotka, Fabian
Ozga, Ann-Kathrin
Palm, Christoph
Pérez Garriga, Ariadna
Plata, Christopher
Plaumann, Markus
Pobiruchin, Monika
Prasser, Fabian
Prokosch, Hans-Ulrich
Przysucha, Mareike
Puladi, Behrus
Rauch, Geraldine
Reimer, Niklas
Reinecke, Ines
Rheinländer, Sophia
Röder, Ingo
Röhrig, Rainer

Rüther, Alric
Sauerbrei, Willi
Sauermann, Stefan
Schemmann, Ulrike
Scherag, André
Schirrmeister, Wiebke
Schmidt, Carsten Oliver
Schmidtmann, Irene
Schmitt, Jochen
Schmücker, Paul
Schreiweis, Björn
Schug, Stephan
Schulte-Coerne, Jonas
Schulze, Mareike
Schuppert, Andreas
Schüttler, Christina
Schwartze, Jonas
Sedlmayr, Brita
Sedlmayr, Martin
Seggewies, Christof
Seifert, Sascha
Sellemann, Björn
Setphan, Astrid
Sohrabi, Keywan
Speer, Ronald
Spicher, Nicolai
Spreckelsen, Cord
Staemmler, Martin
Stang, Andreas
Stausberg, Jürgen
Stein, Markus
Stenzhorn, Holger
Stöhr, Mark R.
Stolpe, Susanne
Storf, Holger
Strahwald, Brigitte
Strauch, Konstantin
Thate, Stefan
Thewes, Dustin
Thun, Sylvia
Tiews, Sven
Timmer, Antje
Toddenroth, Dennis
Triefenbach, Lucas
Truhn, Daniel
Twardella, Dorothee
Ückert, Frank
Ulrich, Hannes
Varghese, Julian

Viehmann, Anja
Vogel, Stefan
Volmerg, Julia S.
Vomweg, Toni
von Dincklage, Falk
Waltemath, Dagmar
Weinert, Lina
Weiß, Christel
Wiedekopf, Joshua
Wienströer, Jan
Wiesner, Martin
Winter, Alfred

Wolf, Ivo
Wolf, Klaus-Hendrik
Wolfien, Markus
Wolkenhauer, Olaf
Wolkewitz, Martin
Wübbeler, Markus
Zapf, Antonia
Zeleke, Atinkut Alamirrew
Zenker, Sven
Zierk, Jakob
Zoch, Michele
Zowalla, Richard

Contents

German Medical Data Sciences 2022 - Future Medicine
R. Röhrig et al. (Eds.)
doi:10.3233/SHTI220797

Development of a Knowledge Base for Chronic Wound Management Using the Decision Model & Notation

Alain FRAYNAL[a,b,1] and Stefan VOGEL[c]

[a]*Medical Informatics and Technology, UMIT - Tirol Private University for Health Sciences, Hall in Tirol, Austria*
[b]*Digital & Automation, Siemens Healthineers, Vienna, Austria*
[c]*Department of Medical Informatics, University Medical Center Göttingen, Germany*

Abstract. Chronic wounds have significant impacts on patient health-related quality of life (HRQoL) and the healthcare expenditures. Various complex decision-making scenarios arise from wound management. Clinical decision-making systems (CDSS) can assist in relieving healthcare providers in these complex decision-making processes and improve the quality of care. In our study, we used the Decision Model & Notation (DMN) standard as a knowledge representation format to implement a knowledge base for chronic wound material recommendation in phase-based therapy. The resulting decision model is theoretically consistent and sustainable. With this study, we also emphasized the need of a semantic interoperability framework. This opens further research possibilities regarding the improvement of the model and the interest of DMN for decision models in clinical fields.

Keywords. Clinical Decision Support Systems, Wound & Injuries, Knowledge Bases, Knowledge Management, Decision Model & Notation

1. Introduction

Clinical Decision Support Systems (CDSS) are tools, which are supposed to assist healthcare providers in dealing with complex clinical decision [1]. A field to develop and explore the potential benefit of CDSS is the one of chronic wound dressing in a phase-based treatment. Wound healing process "consists of four sequential and partially intertwined stages, hemostasis, inflammation, proliferation, and tissue remodeling" [2], [3]. A chronic wound is a wound which is not completely healed after a long time (depending on the publication, this time is stated from four weeks to three months [4]). The increased healing time of chronic wounds is usually due to complex biological processes that correlate with disruption within the four phases of wound healing. A wound has direct and indirect consequences on affected patients and the society [5]. At first, the health-related quality of life (HRQoL) is reduced because it generally decreases their autonomy in addition to decreasing the physical and / or psychological conditions.

---

[1] Corresponding Author, Alain FRAYNAL, Medical Informatics and Technology, UMIT - Tirol Private University for Health Sciences, Eduard-Wallnöfer-Zentrum 1, 6060 Hall in Tirol, Austria / Digital & Automation, Siemens Healthineers, Siemensstraße 90, 1210 Vienna, Austria; E-mail: alain.fraynal@siemens-healthineers.com

This value is "the value assigned to duration of life as modified by the impairments, functional states, perceptions, and social opportunities that are influenced by disease, injury, treatment, or policy." of the patients. The extension of the duration of the healing process may also affect the patient incomes and / or their healthcare expenses, due to potential repetitive sick leaves and hospitalizations, when it is not caused by a subsequent incapacity (for example, related to an amputation) or an early retirement. For the society, the healing process involves many healthcare professionals from the diagnosis, the treatment and the follow-up; the related costs have an important impact, representing 1 to 5.5% of the total healthcare expenditures (depending on the country and the chosen publications) [5]. Chronic wounds and their financial impact are so important that they are sometimes described as an epidemy due to their high incidence rate (in its epidemiologic meaning) [3], [6]. On the other hand, the selection of wound care material rises to a complex decision scenario due to the fact that the caregiver has a variety of causalities, conditions and options to involve in the decision-making process.

At least one CDSS, which deals with chronic wounds, is the PosiThera project [7], [8]. The research group already implemented a prototype for chronic wound management for the decision-making process diagnosis to treatment. It was developed according to two inference methodologies to compare the benefits and drawbacks of both methods and to choose the one, which would be the most adapted to the project framework. The project implementation and analysis work helped to define the standards, which would be used for the solution itself.

Our study focuses on the research question if the Decision Model & Notation (DMN) of the Object Management Group [9]–[11] would be appropriate to model the chronic wound knowledge in phase-based treatment.

The DMN standard was developed to be the language, notation and knowledge representation format for business decisions and rules. It is one knowledge representation approach which is human interpretable and explainable. Hence, it could be a good candidate to support guideline formalization in the preliminary phase to CDSS development.

There are other knowledge representation formats like HL7 Arden Syntax, petri nets and openEHR GDL. The similarities between the HL7 Arden Syntax and other knowledge representation formats were demonstrated in other study works [7] like and might make the translation from one format to another easy to perform.

Moreover, DMN can be combined with two other standards:

- the Business Process Model and Notation (BPMN) for business process representation,
- and the Case Management Model and Notation (CMMN) for business cases representation.

In such a combination, it is possible to have a BPMN or a CMMN diagram which refers to a DMN diagram. As the other knowledge representation formats are limited to decision modeling, DMN presents a clear advantage for the development of easy knowledge exchanges in business in general and in healthcare for clinical decision-making and clinical workflows.

2. Methods

2.1. DMN standard

The DMN standard includes several fundamental definitions and representations which define the framework of decision-making modeling [10], [11].

A "decision" is the action of choosing an option among several possibilities. The "input" data are the variables to be considered in the decision-making situation. The "output" is the chosen option. The "decision logic" defines how the input data drive to the output value using logic.

In DMN formalism, these objects are depicted in a form of a flow diagram which is called "Decision Requirement Diagram" (DRD). In the DRD, the decision is displayed as a rectangle box, Inputs represented as horizontal "cartouche" symbols. Outputs are part of the decision box and has no representative icon. When an element requires information from another one, this "information requirement" is depicted with a solid line and a solid arrowhead which points at the information "requester". Elements of a DRD can be group informally thanks to a group which is represented by a rounded corner rectangle drawn with a solid dashed line.

The standard includes additional elements, but this publication will focus on these fundamentals elements which are the core of the decision modeling.

2.2. Modeling methods

In this study, we used DMN to model the human decision-making in the wound material selection in a phase-based treatment [9]–[11].

Following the steps of Boxwala et al. (2011) [12] which are the unstructured layer, the semi-structured layer, the structured layer and the executable layer, we used a semi-structured guideline which was created through a documentation analysis of the scientific literature. The requirements for an automated decision-making of wound material choice in the form of recommendations was directly waterfalled from the obtained guideline.

Using defined concepts in the DMN standard, it was possible to start modeling the decision-making. The first step was to define the concerned situation in which one or several decisions are needed. This situation can often be described by a question to be answered according to information (given as input data) and the decision logic.

In our case, we concentrated on the decision problem to select the adequate wound material based on contextual wound case information. As inputs, we followed the TIME assessment method (Tissue, Infection, Moisture imbalance, and Edge advancement) [13], [14]. TIME was developed by a wound care consensus group and provides an assessment framework which got high adoption and usage levels amongst healthcare professionals. We defined the outputs as the recommended materials and technics, the retention time, the potential counterindications and additional information which are relevant for the material usage. The materials and technics included different types of dressings, compresses, foams, cream, gels, compression and cleansing technics. For the decision logic, DMN provides three possibilities: literal expressions which can be formal or executable, invocations which list for each defined parameter its corresponding expression, or decision tables.

We to use the decision table method which allowed us to map multiple input values with the corresponding output value in an easy human readable way. As knowledge sources, we used the mentioned rule base in the form of a semi-structured guideline, the associated glossary (the aim of this glossary will be discussed later in this article) and the literature source on which the rule base was created.

To formalize our model, we chose the academic platform of Signavio Process Manager solution [15].

3. Results

We created the modeling with the different element insertion based on the rule base, which could be seen as a wound assessment "questionnaire" with its criteria (each of them associated to a value set). The criteria for patient and wound characterization were set as 17 inputs for the decision (Figure 1).

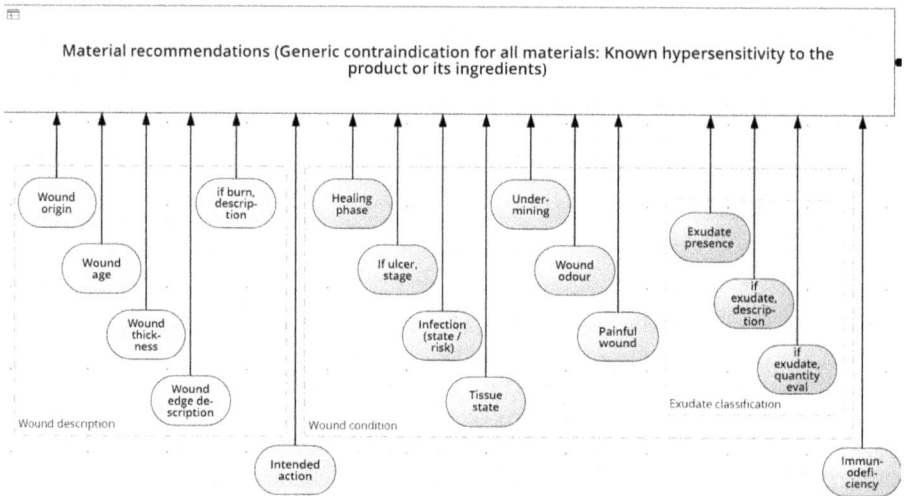

Figure 1. Decision Requirement Diagram of the DMN model for chronic wound material recommendation

The model was complemented by 2 knowledge sources:

- the wound glossary and classifications which was built for this study [16],
- the wound material tables as annexes of the eighth edition of "Moderne Wundversorgung", from Kerstin Protz & Jan Hinnerk Timm (2016) [17].

Fifteen of the inputs were informally grouped in two groups and one "sub-group" describing categories, which could help to create an input form for healthcare professionals. We implemented the first group as the "Wound description" criteria with its origin, its age, its thickness, the description of its edges and its classification if it is a burn. We defined the other group as the one related to the "Wound condition" with parameters providing the healing phase, the stage of the ulcer (in case it would be one), the infection state and risk, the tissue state, and the presence of undermining, odor and pain. Within this second group, we built up a subgroup aiming for the exudate classification. The two last inputs were kept separated because they described possible additional information respectively about the care and the patient. These two last parameters, which were not grouped but are highly important for wound care are the "Intended action" (which could be for example the wound cleaning or draining) and the immune deficiency which addresses misfunctioning of the immune response (predisposing to infection and certain malignancies). With these fundamentals, the Decision Requirement Diagram (DRD) for the wound material recommendation was created. The result of this construction is represented in **Figure 1**.

The Inputs and Outputs were transcribed directly from the two defined groups of the rule base table data. For some rules, the exclusion of a parameter could be a condition of choice for a wound material. The following combination gives a good example for such situation: If a patient presents a wound with the wound description "*Wound age = Chronic wound*" and the wound conditions "*Healing phase = Proliferative phase*", "*Tissue state = no necrotic tissue*" and "*Exudate presence = True*", the recommendation from the rule base would be "*Polyurethane foam dressing / Wound gauze with NOSF (nano-oligosaccharide factor)*". In such a case, the exclusion of a parameter was transcribed with the expression "NOT" (*Criterion A => NOT value X*).

The chosen hit policy could only be a multiple hit policy, because several materials could be recommended for certain combinations of input parameters. Theoretically, the policies "**C**ollect" (C) and "**R**ule order" (R) could be chosen, but the C hit policy would need to be used without an operator ("+", "<", ">", or "#") to get a list of outputs. The hit policy "**O**utput order" (O) could not fit because of the choice to have some of the outputs ("Contraindications" and "Additional information") with text domain (data expressed in natural language) with no value sets. Indeed, no value set caused an impossibility to order the result according to the order in the value set. Before choosing between the two possible policies, it was decided to perform tests to define the most appropriated setup.

When choosing the hit policy, another factor had to be taken into consideration: the completeness of the inputs. In a "*Complete*" decision table, all possible inputs must be considered in the decision table. So, we aimed for the configuration with incomplete data input (option "*Incomplete*") to address real world decision scenarios in which some information might be unknown and/or not filled in by the users.

4. Discussion

4.1. DMN modeling

Through the performed modeling, we managed to show that DMN was appropriate to model the chronic wound material recommendation rule base. A decision table, which was the "heart" of the defined model could be derived for the rule base. The resulting Decision Requirement Graph (DRG) had no decision network but had an important size due to the important number of inputs (17 inputs for 1 Decision element). As we tried to represent the wound assessment process done by professionals, further studies should consider fracturing the model into decision fragments through an iterative process in collaboration with healthcare professionals

The fact Signavio Process Manager only supports DMN version 1.1 [10], [18] could also have been a problem, because the latest version of DMN is the version 1.3 [11]. However, when comparing the two versions, it was shown that this had no impact on the study work, because the changes over the different versions were not on the used level and specifications.

With the DMN model and its decision table, the resulting recommendations are theoretically consistent and sustainable. The Signavio solution enforces this theoretical possibility as it provides easy access to all parameters and rules can be added and/or updated. A test campaign is the obvious next step for the study to check and improve the decision model.

Moreover, Wasylewicz et al. (2018) [19] stated the interests of applying a validation strategy. In any software development and implementation, the validation of the components is a standard and obvious part of those processes. This does not only help to search and solve failures, but it also participates to the software quality in terms of reliability, sustainability, and consistency [20].

4.2. Semantic interoperability

The variation in the perception and knowledge representation among people is at the same time a strength and a weakness for the knowledge communication [21]. In the scientific literature, all publications, be it articles, reports or books, are written in natural language and contain a glossary listing the terms used in the concerned specialty field.

It seems it is particularly the case for the clinical field of chronic wound. In 2018, Kyaw et al. wrote an article which pointed at the absence of a clear and unique definition for the term "chronic wound" [4]. They concluded their review emphasizing two aspects: on one hand, a unique common definition would help to improve wound management. On the other hand, the related guidelines and a "scoring system" based on the patient info and the clinical case would strengthen the diagnosis and the care quality in a multidisciplinary team.

We faced those difficulties and benefits of the implementation of such a semantic normalization work. Due to the needed multi-disciplinary for wound treatment, several scientific societies provide such glossaries. Hence, no standardized terms and definitions were found. This increased the difficulty to select and apply a "specialty-neutral" term and definition set. We used a dedicated glossary for our study but ideally, we should have used a nomenclature which could both be validated by healthcare professionals. In that regard, establishing the mapping of a dataset for wound routine care (which was obtained through a national consensus) [22] with SNOMED CT [23] would be very interesting but would require a significant time frame.

5. Conclusion

With this study, we created a decision model as a rule base for wound material recommendations, and we managed to represent it in the DMN standard [9]–[11], using the knowledge extraction from a medical education book (Protz & Trimm (2016) [17]. The resulting Decision Requirement Diagram included one Decision element and the associated decision table was directly derived from the rule base. This application of the standard confirmed its relevancy to the healthcare sector. It opened consequently the possibility for a better and more transparent exchange of the Decision models for the chronic wound treatment clinical use case.

Concerning the used value sets, the natural language expression allows too much interpretation possibilities and misunderstandings. We also took into account that wound care involves many healthcare specialties. For these reasons, we used a dedicated glossary and classification set because of a time perspective but keeping in mind that the ideal solution would be to use the SNOMED CT nomenclature in association with a glossary issued thanks to a clinical expert consensus [21], [22].

For future research studies, the rule base assessment should be considered in the global modeling work. The model should not only be further tested but also be assessed. Indeed, the tests and assessments of the rules would increase the trust the users could have in the model as well as its level of reliability, sustainability, and consistency. Moreover, Shortliffe et al. (2018), cited by Montani & Striani (2019) [23], mentioned that any recommendation should be understandable by user. Even if our rule base was built on evidence-based literature, creating an assessment indicator inspired by PRISMA meta-analysis method or AMSTAR 2 method could be a solution to improve the transparency and explainability [23] of the rule base. Through this approach, the idea would be to provide a rational and evidence-based evaluation of each recommendation in regards of the clinical researches which were realized for the associated wound material. This knowledge base check is mentioned in an ongoing study as part of the CDSS lifecycle [24] and would help to minimize the risks and to increase the quality of the CDSS development. This approach might also be interesting to support the scrutiny approach mentioned in the Medical Device Regulation for the conformity assessment of some of the class III and class IIb devices (Section 2, Article 55).

Contributions of the authors

AF and SV did the Work Conception, AF created the knowledge base and wrote the Manuscript. SV did the substantial revision of the manuscript. All authors have approved the manuscript as submitted and accept responsibility for the scientific integrity of the work.

Conflict of Interest

The authors declare that there is no conflict of interest.

References

[1]   J. A. Osheroff *et al.*, "Improving Outcomes with Clinical Decision Support: An Implementer's Guide," *Improving Outcomes with Clinical Decision Support*, Feb. 2012, doi: 10.4324/9780367806125.

[2]   X. Zhang, W. Shu, Q. Yu, W. Qu, Y. Wang, and R. Li, "Functional Biomaterials for Treatment of Chronic Wound," *Frontiers in Bioengineering and Biotechnology*, vol. 8, no. June, pp. 1–15, 2020, doi: 10.3389/fbioe.2020.00516.

[3]   M. B. Dreifke, A. A. Jayasuriya, and A. C. Jayasuriya, "Current wound healing procedures and potential care," *Materials Science and Engineering C*, vol. 48, pp. 651–662, 2015, doi: 10.1016/j.msec.2014.12.068.

[4]   B. M. Kyaw, K. Järbrink, L. Martinengo, J. Car, K. Harding, and A. Schmidtchen, "Need for improved definition of 'chronic wounds' in clinical studies," *Acta Dermato-Venereologica*, vol. 98, no. 1, pp. 157–158, 2018, doi: 10.2340/00015555-2786.

[5]   M. Olsson *et al.*, "The humanistic and economic burden of chronic wounds: A systematic review," *Wound Repair and Regeneration*, vol. 27, no. 1, pp. 114–125, 2019, doi: 10.1111/wrr.12683.

[6]   L. Gordis, *Epidemiology, 5th edition*, vol. 62. 2013.

[7]   S. Vogel *et al.*, "Implementation and analysis of two knowledge base approaches for the treatment of chronic wounds," *Studies in Health Technology and Informatics*, vol. 270, pp. 607–612, 2020, doi: 10.3233/SHTI200232.

[8]   (PosiThera Project Consortium), "PosiThera Project - Interprofessional Wound Care," *Simplifier.net*, 2020. https://simplifier.net/PosiThera/~introduction

[9]   (Object Management Group), "Decision Model and Notation™ (DMN™)," *OMG website*, 2021. https://www.omg.org/dmn/index.htm

[10]   (Object Management Group), "Decision Model and Notation version 1.1," *OMG Website*, no. June. 2016. [Online]. Available: https://www.omg.org/spec/DMN/1.1/About-DMN/

[11]   (Object Management Group), "Decision Model and Notation Version 1.3," *OMG Website*, no. January. 2019. [Online]. Available: https://www.omg.org/spec/DMN

[12]   A. A. Boxwala *et al.*, "A multi-layered framework for disseminating knowledge for computer-based decision support," *Journal of the American Medical Informatics Association*, vol. 18, no. SUPPL. 1, pp. 132–139, 2011, doi: 10.1136/amiajnl-2011-000334.

[13]   J. G. Powers, C. Higham, K. Broussard, and T. J. Phillips, "Wound healing and treating wounds Chronic wound care and management," *J Am Acad Dermatol*, vol. 74, no. 4, pp. 607–625, 2016, doi: 10.1016/j.jaad.2015.08.070.

[14]   R. L. Harries, D. C. Bosanquet, and K. G. Harding, "Wound bed preparation: TIME for an update," *International Wound Journal*, vol. 13, pp. 8–14, 2016, doi: 10.1111/iwj.12662.

[15]   (Signavio), "BPM Academic Initiative," *Signavio website*, 2020.

[16]   A. Fraynal and S. Vogel, "Development of a rule base for the recommendation of materials for chronic wound in phase-based treatment using the Decision Model & Notation (DMN)," Hall in Tirol, 2021.

[17]   K. Protz and J. H. Timm, "Wundmaterialen," in *Moderne Wundversorgung*, Urban & Fischer in Elsevier, 2016.

[18]   (Signavio), "Decision Model and Notation (DMN)," *Signavio Process Manager Online Documentation*, 2021. https://documentation.signavio.com/suite/en-us/Content/process-manager/userguide/dmn-intro.htm

[19]   A. T. M. Wasylewicz and A. M. J. W. Scheepers-Hoeks, "Clinical Decision Support Systems," in *Fundamentals of Clinical Data Science*, 2018, pp. 153–169. doi: 10.1007/978-3-319-99713-1.

[20]   A. Spillner, T. Linz, and H. Schaefer, *Software Testing Foundations - A Study Guide for the Certified Tester Exam*. 2014.

[21]   J. Hüsers, M. Przysucha, M. Esdar, S. M. John, and U. H. Hübner, "Expressiveness of an International Semantic Standard for Wound Care: Mapping a Standardized Item Set for Leg Ulcers to the Systematized Nomenclature of Medicine–Clinical Terms," *JMIR Medical Informatics*, vol. 9, no. 10, p. e31980, Oct. 2021, doi: 10.2196/31980.

[22]   K. Heyer *et al.*, "Nationaler Konsens zu Wunddokumentation beim Ulcus cruris," *Der Hautarzt*, vol. 68, no. 9, pp. 740–745, Sep. 2017, doi: 10.1007/s00105-017-4011-7.

[23]   S. Montani and M. Striani, "Artificial Intelligence in Clinical Decision Support: a Focused Literature Survey," *IMIA Yearbook of medical informatics*, vol. 28, no. 1, pp. 120–127, 2019, doi: 10.1055/s-0039-1677911.

[24]   J. Richter and S. Vogel, "Illustration of clinical decision support system development complexity," in *Studies in Health Technology and Informatics*, 2020, vol. 272. doi: 10.3233/SHTI200544.

German Medical Data Sciences 2022 - Future Medicine
R. Röhrig et al. (Eds.)

doi:10.3233/SHTI220798

The Interpretation of Verbal Probabilities: A Systematic Literature Review and Meta-Analysis

Hannah VOGEL[a], Sebastian APPELBAUM[a,b], Heidemarie HALLER[c], Thomas OSTERMANN[a,1]

[a] *Department for Psychology and Psychotherapy, Witten/Herdecke University, Alfred Herrhausen-Straße 50, 58448 Witten, Germany*
[b] *Trimberg Research Academy, University of Bamberg, An der Weberei 5, 96047 Bamberg, Germany*
[c] *Department of Internal and Integrative Medicine, Evang. Kliniken Essen-Mitte, Faculty of Medicine, University of Duisburg-Essen, Am Deimelsberg 34a, 45276 Essen, Germany*

Abstract. Introduction: Verbal probabilities such as "likely" or "probable" are commonly used to describe situations of uncertainty or risk and are easy and natural to most people. Numerous studies are devoted to the translation of verbal probability expressions to numerical probabilities. **Methods:** The present work aims to summarize existing research on the numerical interpretation of verbal probabilities. This was accomplished by means of a systematic literature review and meta-analysis conducted alongside the MOOSE-guidelines for meta-analysis of observational studies in epidemiology. Studies were included, if they provided empirical assignments of verbal probabilities to numerical values. **Results:** The literature search identified 181 publications and finally led to 21 included articles and the procession of 35 verbal probability expressions. Sample size of the studies ranged from 11 to 683 participants and covered a period of half a century from 1967 to 2018. In half of the studies, verbal probabilities were delivered in a neutral context followed by a medical context. Mean values of the verbal probabilities range from 7.24% for the term "impossible" up to 94.79% for the term "definite". **Discussion:** According to the results, there is a common 'across-study' consensus of 35 probability expressions for describing different degrees of probability, whose numerical interpretation follows a linear course. However, heterogeneity of studies was considerably high and should be considered as a limiting factor.

Keywords. Verbal probabilities, Meta-analysis, Numerical representation, Systematic review

1. Introduction

Within the last decades, the use and interpretation of verbal probability expressions (VPE) has been intensively investigated from different perspectives such as the field of economics, politics or the health sector [1-5]. VPE are commonly used to describe situations of uncertainty or risk and according to [6] are easy and natural to most people.

---

[1] Thomas Ostermann, Department of Psychology and Psychotherapy, Witten/Herdecke University, Alfred-Herrhausen-Straße 50, 58448 Witten, Germany; E-mail: thomas.ostermann@uni-wh.de.

Brun and Teigen (1988) observed that physicians preferred communicating probabilities verbally whereas their patients rather preferred receiving health-related information numerically [2]. A problem in the transfer of verbal into numerical probabilities is the considerable between-subject variability in the use and interpretations of VPE [1,7]. For example, wide between-subject variations were found for the expression "likely", which was assigned probability estimates ranging from p = .5 to p = .95 [8].

Concurrently, individuals show an internal consistence in the use and interpretation of VPE [9,10]. Dhami and Wallsten (2005) linked those findings and argued, that individuals have a stable lexicon of VPE, which however may differ considerably among individuals [7]. Still, interpersonal consensus regarding the probabilistic meaning of an expression may be derived by examining the rank order of the expression within each lexicon. The authors suggest that expressions or phrases, which are ranked equally, are likely to have similar meanings even though the exact wording differs among individuals. These results are supported in [11], where the authors observed the rank order of a set of 23 VPE to be relatively stable in a British, Hellenic and Malaysian sample. However, the numerical values that were assigned to each VPE turned out to differ considerably between nationalities.

A central concern in the interpretational variability of VPE thus is the danger of communicative misunderstandings [12]. According to [2] most individuals are unaware of both the ambiguity of VPE as well as the variability of VPE interpretations in the general population. Hence, various examinations have focused on providing a translation aid from verbal to numerical probabilities or vice versa [8,9,10,13,14,15].

The current work addresses this translational issue and aims at systematically reviewing and summarizing the existing literature about numerical interpretations of VPE in order to provide an overview of previous research results. In addition to the identification and description of studies involving the numerical interpretation of verbal probabilities, numerical interpretations of frequently examined VPE will be summarized statistically in order to generate a bundled numerical interpretation of each identified VPE.

2. Methods

This systematic review and meta-analysis was conducted alongside the guidelines for meta-analysis of observational studies in epidemiology (MOOSE) [16]. The following electronic databases were searched from their inception to 2020 independently by two authors: Psychological and Behavioral Science Collection (PBSC), PubMed, PsycArticles and CINAHL. The literature search was constructed around the search term 'verbal probabilities' and adapted for each database as necessary. Furthermore, reference lists of identified original articles and reviews were searched manually for further relevant articles.

Articles were included, if they studied empirical assignments of verbal probabilities to numerical values (from 0% to 100% or 0 to 1). Articles including numerical interpretation of verbal probabilities using another numerical format (e.g. five-point Likert scales or membership functions) were not included. Expressions such as 'rare', 'commonly' or 'often' referring to frequencies rather than probabilities and were not considered in the current work. Furthermore, only studies published in German, English, or Spanish were considered. Book chapters and unpublished studies were excluded.

Included studies were analyzed regarding the year of publication, country, method of capturing the probability interpretation, numerical format, and the thematic context of the verbal probability assessment. Furthermore, the total amount of VPE examined in the studies and identified mean values, standard deviations as well as sample size for each study were extracted.

To review expressions that are used with a certain consensus, only VPE that were interpreted in at least four investigations were further processed. A meta-analysis for each VPE using the random effects model was calculated by R package 'meta' [17]. In cases of missing standard deviations, they were calculated by the average standard deviation of the remaining studies within the corresponding VPE. Missing sample sizes were substituted using the median of reported sample sizes of the remaining studies.

3. Results

The database search revealed 163 articles. Reviewing reference lists of identified articles led to the consideration of 18 further articles. After removal of duplicates, 87 articles were excluded by screening title and abstracts. Full texts of the remaining 49 records were reviewed and assessed for eligibility. Further articles had to be excluded as the respective full-text was not available, published in a different language, had a different numerical format, or did not present detailed results for meta-analysis. The selection process is illustrated in figure 1.

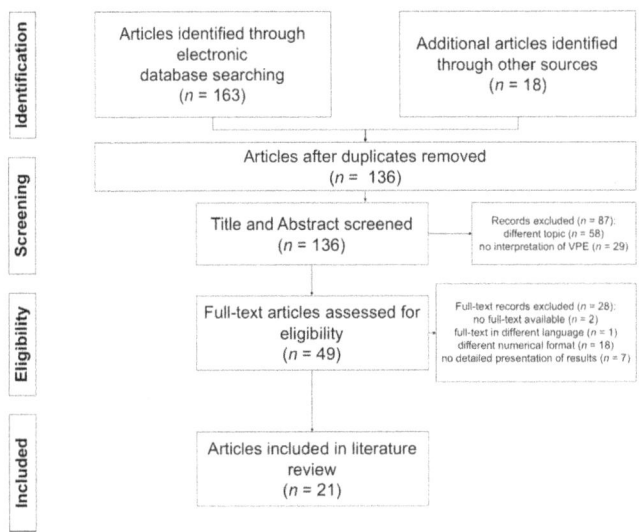

Fig 1. Flow chart of the literature selection process. n = here: number of articles; VPE = verbal probability expressions.

Table 1 provides an overview of the 21 included studies. Sample size of the studies ranged from 11 to 683 participants (Mean: 111.75 Median: 70) and covered a period of half a century from 1967 to 2018. Origin of the studies was mixed with n=10 studies from the USA followed by the UK (n=3) and Norway (n=2). Most of the studies (n=11) used a population of students or medical staff (n=4). Only one study asked a sample of patients. The VPE in half of the studies (n=10) were delivered in a neutral context followed by a medical context (n=7).

Table 1. Overview of the included studies.

First Author	Year	Origin	N	Sample	Context
Bergenstrom [18]	2003	UK/USA	87	Medical students	Medical
Brun [2]	1988	Norway	16	Psychology students	Neutral
Budescu [9]	1985	USA	32	Psychology students	Neutral
Chee [11]	2006	Malaysia	32	Mixed (mainly students)	Neutral
Cohn [4]	2009	Mexico/USA	263	Mixed (mainly students)	Medical
Damrosch [19]	1983	USA	70	Female nurses	Medical
Hamm [13]	1991	USA	140	Psychology students	Neutral
Hobby [20]	2000	UK	11	Physicians	Medical
Honda [21]	2006	Japan	137	Students	Gambling
Honda [21]	2006	Japan	67	Students	Gambling
Juhanchich [22]	2013	USA	84	Workers	Neutral
Kong [12]	1986	USA	n/a	Medical staff	Medical
Lichtenstein [15]	1967	USA	188	Employees	Neutral
Ostermann [23]	2018	Germany	683	Mixed (mainly students)	Neutral
Reagan [8]	1989	USA	115	Psychology students	Neutral
Shying [24]	2013	HK, MYS, SGP	55	Auditors	Neutral
Sutherland [25]	1991	Canada	100	Cancer patients	Medical
Tavana [26]	1997	USA	30	Financial experts	Banking
Teigen [27]	2001	Norway	20	Psychology students	Job offer
Teixera [5]	2009	Portugal	35	Auditors	Neutral
Villejoubert [28]	2009	UK	70	Medical staff	Medical

Statistical analyses were based on the following 35 VPE, which had been examined by at least four included articles: almost certain (n = 7), almost impossible (n = 5), certain (n = 7), chance (n = 4), definite (n = 4), doubtful (n = 4), good chance (n = 6), highly improbable (n = 6), highly probable (n = 8), impossible (n = 5), improbable (n = 8), likely (n = 18), maybe (n = 6), not certain (n = 7), not likely (n = 4), not possible (n = 5), not probable, (n = 4), perhaps (n = 4), possible (n = 22), possibly (n = 4), probable (n = 19), quite likely (n = 7), quite probable (n = 4), quite unlikely (n = 9), reasonable assurance (n = 4), reasonably certain (n = 4), reasonably possible (n = 4), remote (n = 4), somewhat doubtful (n = 4), uncertain (n = 11), unlikely (n = 14), very likely (n = 8), very probable (n = 10), very unlikely (n = 10), virtually certain (n = 4). Figures 2 to 4 provide forest plots for the VPE "unlikely", "uncertain" and "likely".

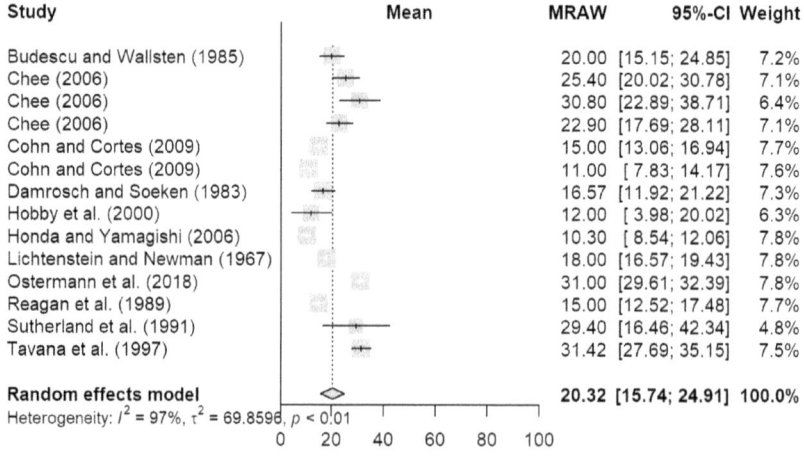

Fig 2. Forest plot of the meta-analysis of the expression "unlikely" from (MRAW: Raw Mean).

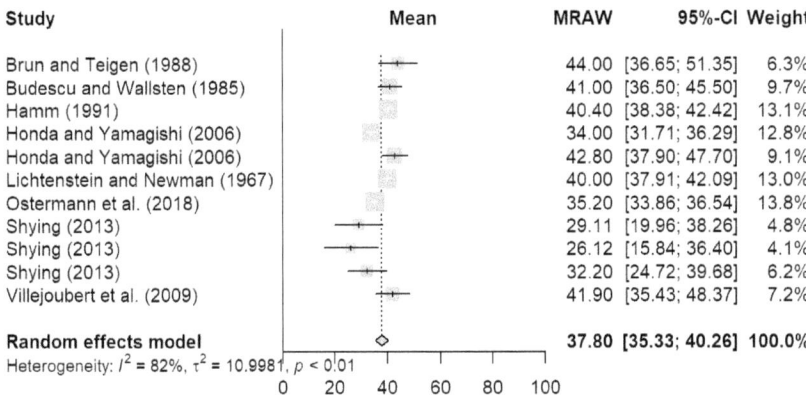

Fig 3. Forest plot of the meta-analysis of the expression "uncertain" (MRAW: Raw Mean).

Between-study heterogeneity for each was highly significant in 29 out of 35 cases except for the expressions "remote" ($I^2 = 0.00$; $\tau^2 = 0.00$; p = 0.604), "somewhat doubtful" ($I^2 = 2.60$; $\tau^2 = 0.68$; p = 0.380), "reasonably possible" ($I^2 = 15.40$; $\tau^2 = 2.52$; p = 0.315), "reasonable assurance" ($I^2 = 40.70$; $\tau^2 = 3.70$; p = 0.168), "reasonably certain" ($I^2 = 3.30$; $\tau^2 = 0.21$; p = 0.376) and "virtually certain" ($I^2 = 64.80$; $\tau^2 = 11.82$; p = 0.036).

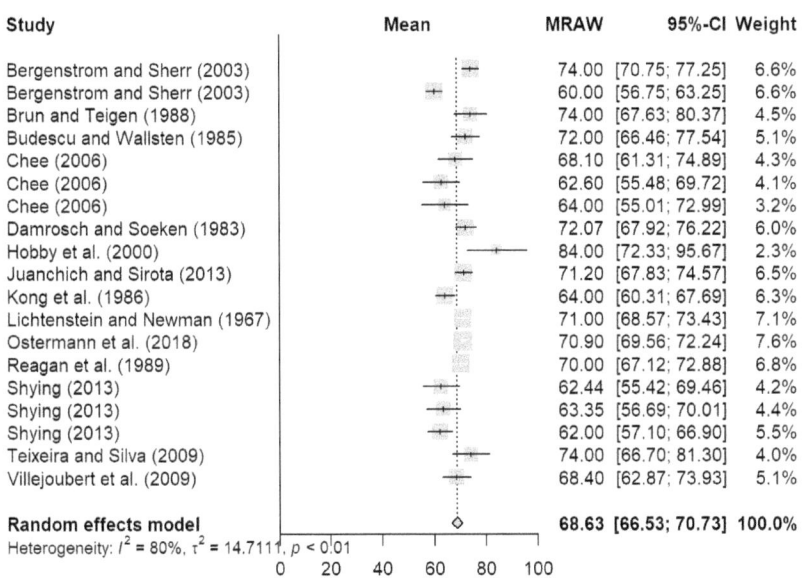

Fig 4. Forest plot of the meta-analysis of the expression "likely" (MRAW: Raw Mean).

The complete results of the random effects model for all VPEs are provided in Fig. 5, in which the weighted mean with 95% confidence interval is displayed.

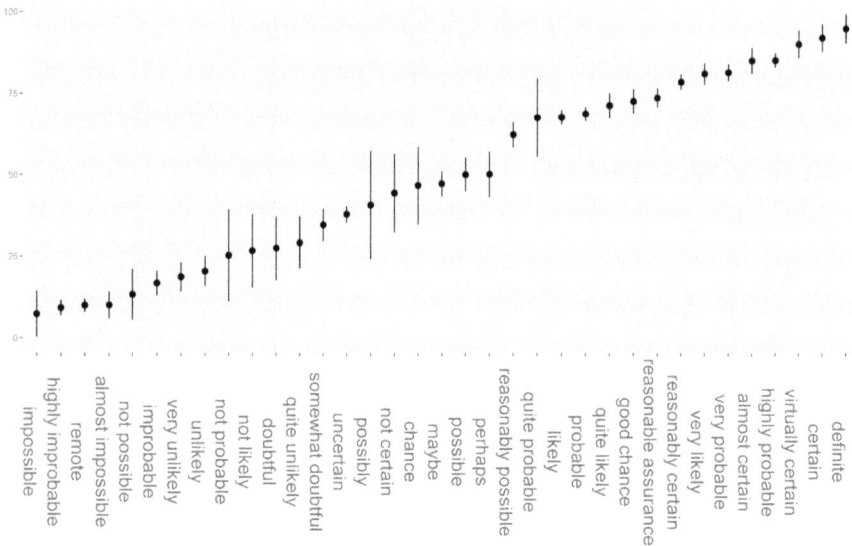

Fig 5. Averaged mean values of 35 verbal probability expressions across the respective studies; error bars denote the 95% confidence intervals.

Mean values of the VPE interpretations range from 7.24% (SE: 3.58) for the VPE "impossible" up to 94.79% (SE: 2.26) for the VPE "definite". The greatest leap can be found between the expressions "perhaps" (M: 50.05; SE: 3.57) and "reasonably possible" (M: 62.22; SE: 1.98). Nevertheless, the 35 expressions are apparently linear distributed across the continuum between 0 and 100%.

4. Discussion

This work aimed at systematically reviewing the existing literature on the interpretation of verbal probabilities. Studies including a numerical interpretation of VPE were included and further analyzed. A large number of expressions are compound words, consisting of a central expression of probability accompanied by a further expression used to describe the degree of probability more specifically such as barely possible, entirely possible or faintly possible. This results in innumerable differentiations of probability expressions compared to the central expression, for example 'possible'.

The extracted set of 35 VPE can thus be cautiously considered a common 'across-study' lexicon of verbal probability terms, and is evenly distributed within the range between 7.24% (impossible) up to 94.79% (definite). The present results provide strong evidence for VPE interpretations behaving in a linear rather than somehow logistic way.

Although this meta-analysis has its strength in synthesizing more than 40 years of research in numerical estimations of verbal probabilities, it also has several limitations. Firstly, we only searched for the term "verbal probabilities". Although this is the most common term in this field of research, we might have missed literature by using only a single term. We also decided against a risk of bias assessment, which normally attributes issues like "random sequence generation", "allocation concealment", "blinding" or "selective reporting" which is an important issue in RCTs. Our analysis however only deals with surveys without control groups and blinding and thus we cannot give information on a risk of bias. Another major limitation is given by the heterogeneity of studies, indicated by means of I^2 and τ^2, which is considerably high with 29 out of 35 comparisons reaching statistical significance. Including and comparing heterogeneous studies is one of the main criticisms regarding the method of a meta-analysis casually known as the 'apples and oranges problem' [29]. We however decided to include the studies in this investigation, as we just aimed at summing up existing numerical interpretations on VPE. The inclusion criteria set out above served the purpose to identify studies with comparable research questions and methodology.

A further limitation of the present meta-analysis is the combination of studies from different research contexts as well as uncontextualized investigations. Since previous examinations demonstrated the context of VPE to influence their numerical interpretation [1,2] future research should combine investigations using comparable contexts or address different contexts in subgroup analyses.

5. Conclusion

Our results systematically reviewed the existing literature on VPE and revealed, that a considerable amount of studies addresses the numerical interpretation of VPE; however, using different numerical formats. Considering studies using the format of percentages or probabilities leads to the identification of a broad variety of different probability expressions that were apparently linear distributed within the range from 0% to 100%. According to our results, there is a common 'across-study' consensus of 35 VPE for describing different degrees of probability, whose numerical interpretation follows a linear course as discussed in [23].

6. Conflict of Interest

The authors state that they have no conflict of interests.

7. Author's contribution

Conceptualization: Thomas Ostermann, Hannah Vogel, Heidemarie Haller; Methodology: Thomas Ostermann, Sebastian Appelbaum; Formal analysis: Sebastian Appelbaum; Writing – original draft: Hannah Vogel, Thomas Ostermann; Writing – review & editing: Thomas Ostermann, Heidemarie Haller, Sebastian Appelbaum, Hannah Vogel; Supervision: Thomas Ostermann.

References

[1] R. Beyth-Marom. How probable is probable? A numerical translation of verbal probability expressions. *Journal of Forecasting*, (1982), **1(3)**, 257–269.
[2] W. Brun, K.H. Teigen. Verbal probabilities: ambiguous, context-dependent, or both? *Organizational Behavior and Human Decision Processes*, (1988), **41**, 390–404.

[3] D.V. Budescu, T.M. Karelitz, T.S. Wallsten. Predicting the directionality of probability words from their membership functions. *Journal of Behavioral Decision Making*, (2003), **16(3)**, 159–180.

[4] L. Cohn, M. Cortes. Quantifying risk: verbal probability expressions in Spanish and English. *American Journal of Health Behavior*, (2009), **33(3)**, 244–255.

[5] C. Teixeira, A.F. Silva. The interpretation of verbal probability expressions used in the IAS/IFRS: some Portuguese evidence. *Polytechnical Studies Review*, (2009), **7(12)**, 57–73.

[6] A. C. Zimmer. A model for the interpretation of verbal predictions. *International Journal of Man-Machine Studies*, (1984), **20(1)**, 121–134.

[7] M. K. Dhami, T. S. Wallsten. Interpersonal comparison of subjective probabilities: toward translating linguistic probabilities. *Memory & Cognition*, (2005), **33(6)**, 1057–1068.

[8] R. T. Reagan, F. Mosteller, C. Youtz. Quantitative meanings of verbal probability expressions. *Journal of Applied Psychology*, (1989), **74(3)**, 433–442.

[9] D. V. Budescu, T. S. Wallsten. Consistency in interpretation of probabilistic phrases. *Organizational Behavior and Human Decision Processes*, (1985), **36(3)**, 391–405.

[10] D. A. Clark. Verbal uncertainty expressions: a critical review of two decades of research. *Current Psychology: Research & Reviews*, (1990), **9(3)**, 203–235.

[11] C. S. Chee. "In-Isolation" study on verbal uncertainty expressions. *Proceedings of the 2nd IMT-GT Regional Conference on Mathematics, Statistics and Applications,* (2006), University Sains Malaysia, Penang.

[12] A. Kong, G. O. Barnett, F. Mosteller, C. Youtz. How medical professionals evaluate expressions of probability. *The New England Journal of Medicine*, (1986), **315(12)**, 740–744.

[13] R. M. Hamm. Selection of verbal probabilities: a solution for some problems of verbal probability expression. *Organizational Behavior and Human Decision Processes*, (1991), **48(2)**, 193–223.

[14] C. Witteman, S. Renooij. Evaluation of a verbal–numerical probability scale. International *Journal of Approximate Reasoning*, (2003), **33(2)**, 117–131.

[15] S. Lichtenstein, J. R. Newman. Empirical scaling of common verbal phrases associated with numerical probabilities. *Psychonomic Science*, (1967), **9(10)**, 563–564.

[16] D. F. Stroup, J. A. Berlin, S. C. Morton, I. Olkin, G. D. Williamson, D. Rennie, D. Moher, B. J. Becker, T. A. Sipe, S. B. Thacker. Meta-analysis of observational studies in epidemiology: a proposal for reporting. *JAMA*, (2000), **283(15)**, 2008-2012.

[17] S. Balduzzi, G. Rücker, G. Schwarzer. How to perform a meta-analysis with R: A practical tutorial. *Evidence-Based Mental Health*, (2019), **22(4)**, 153–160.

[18] A. Bergenstrom, L. Sherr. The effect of order of presentation of verbal probability expressions on numerical estimates in a medical context. *Psychology, Health & Medicine*, (2003), **8(4)**, 391–398.

[19] S. P. Damrosch, K. Soeken. Communicating probability in clinical reports: Nurses' numerical associations to verbal expressions. *Research in Nursing & Health*, (1983), **6(2)**, 85–87.

[20] J. L. Hobby, B. D. Tom, C. Todd, P.W. Bearcroft, A. K. Dixon. Communication of doubt and certainty in radiological reports. *The British Journal of Radiology*, (2000), **73(873)**, 999–1001.

[21] H. Honda, K. Yamagishi. Directional verbal probabilities: Inconsistencies between preferential judgments and numerical meanings. *Experimental Psychology*, (2006), **53(3)**, 161–170.

[22] M. Juanchich, M. Sirota. Do people really say it is "likely" when they believe it is only "possible"? Effect of politeness on risk communication. *Quarterly Journal of Experimental Psychology*, (2013), **66(7)**, 1268–1275.

[23] T. Ostermann, H. Vogel, S. Appelbaum. Verbal probabilities: linear or logistic? - A regression analysis approach. *Studies in Health Technology and Informatics*, (2018), **253**, 117–121.

[24] M. Shying. Auditors interpretations of "in-isolation" verbal probability expressions: A cross-national study. In M. Kennelley: The Influence of Environmental and Cultural Factors in International Accounting. Symposium conducted at the American Accounting Associations (AAA) Annual Meeting, Philadelphia. (2013). Available at: https://www.sec.gov/rules/concept/s70400/shying1.htm

[25] H. J. Sutherland, G. A. Lockwood, D. L. Tritchler, F. Sem, L. Brooks, J. E. Till. Communicating probablistic Information to cancer patients: is there 'noise' on the line? *Social Science & Medicine*, (1991), **32(6)**, 725–731.

[26] M. Tavana, D. Kennedy, B. Mohebbi. An Applied Study Using the Analytic Hierarchy Process to Translate Common Verbal Phrases to Numerical Probabilities. *Journal of Behavioral Decision Making*, (1997), **10(2)**, 133–150.

[27] K. H. Teigen. When Equal Chances = Good Chances: Verbal Probabilities and the Equiprobability Effect. *Organizational Behavior and Human Decision Processes*, (2001), **85(1)**, 77–108.

[28] G. Villejoubert, L. Almond, L. Alison. Interpreting claims in offender profiles: the role of probability phrases, base-rates and perceived dangerousness. *Applied Cognitive Psychology*, (2009), **23(1)**, 36–54.

[29] D. Sharpe. Of apples and oranges, file drawers and garbage: why validity issues in meta-analysis will not go away. *Clinical Psychology Review*, (1997), **17(8)**, 881–901.

German Medical Data Sciences 2022 - Future Medicine
R. Röhrig et al. (Eds.)
© 2022 The authors and IOS Press.
This article is published online with Open Access by IOS Press and distributed under the terms
of the Creative Commons Attribution Non-Commercial License 4.0 (CC BY-NC 4.0).
doi:10.3233/SHTI220799

EsteR – A Digital Toolkit for COVID-19 Decision Support in Local Health Authorities

Sonja JÄCKLE[a,1], Rieke ALPERS[a], Lisa KÜHNE[b], Jakob SCHUMACHER[c], Benjamin GEISLER[a] and Max WESTPHAL[a]

[a] *Fraunhofer Institute for Digital Medicine MEVIS, Bremen / Lübeck, Germany*
[b] *Leibniz Institute for Preventive Research and Epidemiology BIPS, Bremen, Germany*
[c] *Local Health Authority Berlin-Reinickendorf, Berlin, Germany*

Abstract. In Germany, the current COVID-19 cases are managed and reported by the local health authorities. The workload of their employees during the pandemic is high, especially in periods of high infection numbers. In this work a decision support toolkit for local health authorities is introduced. A demonstrator web application was developed with the R Shiny framework and is publicly accessible online. It contains five separate tools based on statistical models for specific use cases and corresponding questions of COVID-19 cases and their contacts. The underlying statistical methods have been implemented in a new open-source R package. The toolkit has the potential to support local health authorities' employees in their daily work. A simulated-based validation of the statistical models and a usability evaluation of the demonstrator application in a user study will be carried out in the future.

Keywords. COVID-19, Quarantine, Decision Support Techniques, Public Health, Statistical Models

1. Introduction

The current COVID-19 pandemic is a huge burden for the 378 local health authorities in Germany, which are responsible for managing the COVID-19 cases. Their work includes contacting and informing infected persons to isolate themselves. The local health authorities have to trace contacts of infected persons, record incoming test results from laboratories and order quarantine. In addition, outbreak events must be investigated with special attention. The overall workload of health authorities due to the COVID-19 pandemic is so high that they temporarily prioritize their work towards managing the pandemic [1]. In periods of high infection rates, the local health authorities were not able to trace back contacts of infected persons [2].

Decision support systems can streamline and simplify such processes. For example, in clinics, such tools are already used for diagnosis, triage and prognosis, as well as personalized support for treatment decisions and automated tools for monitoring [3,4]. Moreover, models for predicting the number of COVID-19 infections have been

---

[1] Corresponding Author, Sonja Jäckle, Fraunhofer Institute for Digital Medicine MEVIS, Maria-Goeppert-Straße 3, 23562 Lübeck, Germany; E-mail: sonja.jaeckle@mevis.fraunhofer.de

proposed [5], which allow governments to adapt their regulations to control the pandemic. Network models can be used to analyze the effect of different social distancing scenarios on the spread of COVID 19 [6] and strategies to prevent a second wave [7]. Furthermore, tools for personal usage have been developed, e.g., a COVID-19 aerosol transmission risk calculator [8] to estimate the infection risk for indoor meetings and the microCOVID calculator [9] which allows to assess the infection risk for specific situations or for the whole day.

To the best of our knowledge, there are no tools for the guidance of quarantine and isolation orders at the local level. Most of the local health authorities use SurvNet [10], which is a reporting management software developed and released by the Robert-Koch Institute (RKI), and/or SORMAS [11], which is a system for epidemic management. Both software applications allow the management of COVID-19 cases and contacts, but up to now do not include decision support tools or statistical models.

The aim of our project is to support the local health authorities with a decision support web application based on statistical modeling. For this purpose, statistical models have been developed for certain use cases, which are described in section 2. Afterwards, the resulting R package smidm is described, and the web application is illustrated and discussed in section 3 and 4. Finally, the paper ends with section 5 containing conclusions and future work.

2. Methods

In cooperation with the local health authority Berlin-Reinickendorf different use cases and questions were determined. For these problems, tools based on statistical models were developed as decision support. Each tool of the application is explained in more detail.

2.1. Infection period

In this use case, the most likely time point of infection of one or more infected persons is visualized. In a systematic review and meta-analysis in [12] the reported pooled mean and median of the COVID-19 incubation period were 6.3 and 5.4 days, respectively. The most widely used distributions for parametrization of the incubation period were normal and log-normal, but the reported mean and median are not equal. Thus, it was decided to use a log-normal distribution. The needed parameters were directly calculated from the reported mean and median as 1.69 for the mean parameter and 0.55 for the standard deviation parameter. Based on the symptom onset date, the probability of infection in the days before symptom onset is shown in this tool, as well as the high-density regions [13] for 80% and 95%.

Beside one infected person, the tool allows to examine the infection period of several infected persons. Then, the user has to enter all symptom onset dates, and how many persons had their symptom onset on each date. Based on this input, a mixture density $p_{inf}(t)$ is created

$$p_{inf}(t) = \sum_{i=1}^{n_p} w_i \cdot p_{inf_i}(t), \quad w_i = \frac{n_i}{n}, \tag{1}$$

where n is the number of infected persons, n_p is the number of symptom onset dates and $p_{inf_i}(t)$ is the density and n_i the number of persons for the i-th symptom onset date. The resulting mixture density is again a probability density and gives an overview of the possible infection periods of all considered infected persons.

2.2. Illness period

A person infected with COVID-19 is considered and the question is when the infected contacts will show first symptoms. Zhang et al [14] estimated gamma distribution parameters for the serial interval between symptom onsets of infected persons and the symptom onset of infected contacts as 2.39 for the shape and 0.48 for the rate parameter. For our tool, those gamma parameters were used and based on the symptom onset of the infected person the probability of symptom onsets of the infected contacts is displayed together with the 80% and 95% high-density regions.

Furthermore, the tool allows to show the probabilities of symptom onset for the second and third generation of contacts. These probabilities are determined by a convolution of the probability density function of the previous generation with the probability density function for infecting the next generation of contacts. Thereby, the assumption is made that the infection transmissions are independent from contact generation to generation. For gamma distributions, a convolution of two gamma distribution equals the summation of their first parameters, so for each contact generation the model has the gamma distribution

$$p_{ill_g}(t) \sim \Gamma\,(g \cdot \alpha, \beta) \tag{2}$$

where α, β are the shape and the rate parameter for probability distribution, when the infected contacts of an infected person show first symptoms, and g is the considered generation.

In the demonstrator app the probability distributions and their 80% and 95% high-density regions [13] for the first, second and third generation are calculated, and the user can select which one should be shown.

2.3. Infectious period

With this tool, the potentially infectious period can be calculated for an infected person. In literature, an analysis of COVID-19 viral shedding and transmissibility was reported and a gamma distribution for infectious period of cases/patients was estimated based on the symptom onset date [15]. The authors provided an R script from which the shape parameter can be calculated as 20.52 and the rate parameter as 1.60 Based on that, this gamma distribution as well as the 80% and 95% high-density regions [13] are displayed to show when an infected person with symptoms is and was most likely infectious based on the symptom onset date.

For infected persons without symptoms, the period during which the person has to be considered as infectious is calculated according to the regulations of the Robert Koch-Institute (RKI) [16] and visualized. Based on the entered earliest infection date and date of positive testing, the calculated period is visualized on a timeline.

2.4. Infection Spread

The following situation is considered: a group of people has met at a certain event and some of them started to show symptoms in the first days after the event. Assuming that their symptoms are due to an infection at the specific event, the tool gives a worst-case prediction for how many people of the group are expected to be infected and to show symptoms in the following days.

First, two predictions for the total number of symptomatic infections in the group are done: The lognormal density for the incubation time described in 2.1 is used to calculate the percentage of all symptomatic infections to occur up to the last day with an observed illness. Based on the total number of observed illnesses so far, the expected total number of symptomatic infections inside the given group is then determined. In the other approach, the results from Davies et al. [17] are used, who studied the age-dependency of the transmission of COVID-19. For low, medium and high risk the reported 2.5% quantile, mean and 97.5% quantile of the infection rate were averaged over different age groups and multiplied by the corresponding age-specific mean symptom rate (Table 1). The product gives a literature-based prognosis of the setting-specific rate of symptomatic infections inside the group, independent of already observed infections. An absolute value of predicted symptomatic infections is calculated by multiplying this rate with the total group size.

Table 1. Age group-specific infection and symptom rates among infected persons calculated from Extended Data Fig. 4, p. 1218 in [17].

Age Group	Low risk infection rate	Medium risk infection rate	High risk infection rate	Symptom rate
<20	0.26	0.39	0.55	0.25
20-59	0.63	0.81	0.97	0.38
>59	0.63	0.81	0.95	0.66
mixed	0.54	0.71	0.85	0.41

To estimate the worst-case prediction, the maximum of the two predicted numbers of total symptomatic infections is used and split up according to the incubation time density mentioned above to estimate how many people will show symptoms on each of the following days after the last observed illness.

2.5. Risk assessment for group quarantine

In this use case, the following situation is considered: A group met and at least one person was infected. After the contact event, tests (e.g., polymerase chain reaction PCR tests) were performed by part of the group and all test results were negative. With the tool, the probability that no one was infected and that no further cases will occur can be calculated.

The statistical model used for this tool as well as all necessary parameters are described in [18] and has been specified for certain situations such as school classes or children daycare centers, which are the most common use cases in local health authorities. Beside PCR tests, antigen tests can be considered, which have been used more frequently since the beginning of 2021.

3. Results

3.1. R package smidm

All functions needed for the statistical models of each tool were developed in R [19] and have been bundled in the package *statistical modelling for infectious disease management* (smidm). The functions for visualization are not part of the package but are shown in the vignettes. The package smidm is available on Fraunhofer Git repository (https://gitlab.cc-asp.fraunhofer.de/ester/smidm/) for other R users and is published under the BSD-3 license.

3.2. Demonstrator web application

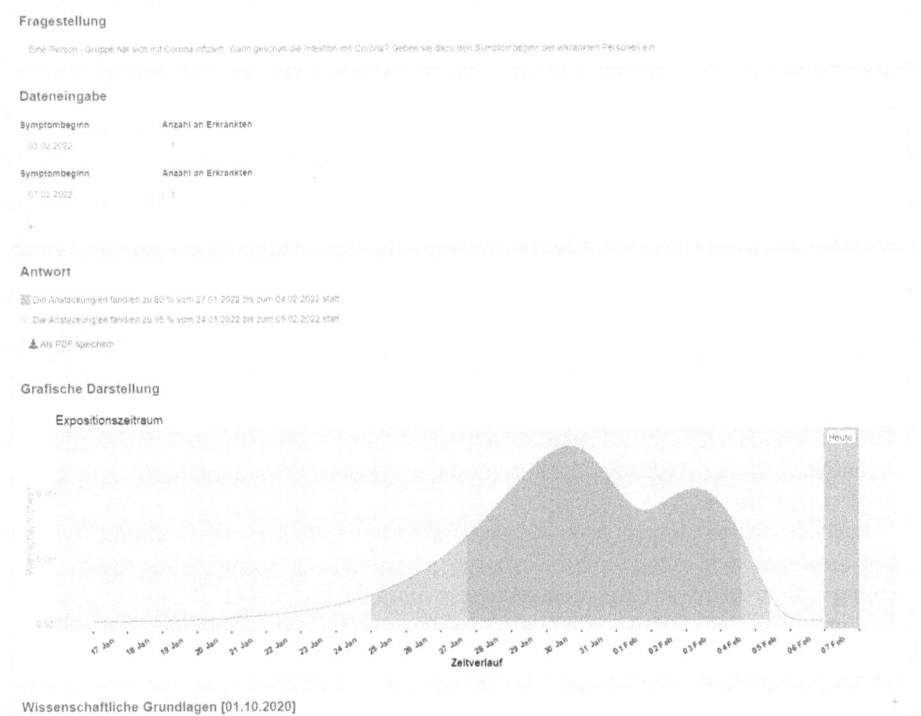

Wissenschaftliche Grundlagen [01.10.2020]

Figure 1. Screenshot of the web application showing the infection period tab for two persons with symptoms onset on 03. and 07. February 2022.

The web application was developed with the R shiny framework [20] and uses the statistical model functions of the smidm package. The demonstrator web application can be accessed at https://ester.fraunhofer.de/. On the starting page, the users get an overview of all existing tools, and whether they apply to single infected persons or to group situations. All tools have the same, consistent structure and layout: the considered situation and question is described, the necessary inputs can be entered, and the answer is given as a text output and a corresponding visualization is shown if applicable. At the bottom, the tool lists the used scientific literature.

The web application has been introduced to employees of the local health authority Berlin-Reinickendorf to detect misunderstandings and to enhance the usability. In the process, the demonstrator was briefly introduced and then given to the employees. They used it for their purposes and shared their feedback with us. This allowed us to conclude how employees use the tools, whether the interface is usable for them, and where usability can be further improved in the application. The results were then used to simplify and restructure the tools and the web application.

A screenshot of the resulting web application showing the infection period tab for two infected persons with symptom onset date on 3. and 7. February 2022 is shown in Figure 1. The considered situation and question of the tab is described briefly and precisely in the first section. The symptom onset dates can be entered with the built-in calendar, further dates can be added and unneeded entries can be removed. Based on the entered inputs, the results are immediately and automatically calculated. In this tab, the text answer simultaneously serves as a legend for the 80% and 95% intervals in the plotted graphs.

4. Discussion

The developed web application can support the daily work of employees at local health authorities, but the benefit of our demonstrator application is limited, because it presumably cannot help overloaded personnel and will not be used by them. Furthermore, the statistical models were developed for specific use cases, where we assumed only information, which typically available for employees at the local health authorities. When cases are reported, no information about the transmission dynamic are available, e.g., whether a super spreading event took place. Hence, our models give a generic view of the transmission dynamics. Until now, no full evaluation of the statistical models has been done and it is not clear how much the employees benefit from using the web application in their daily work. For this purpose, we plan to conduct different simulation studies for validating each statistical model. In addition, a usability study for evaluating the benefit of using the web application for the employees in the local health authorities will be conducted.

Furthermore, parameters from the most recent literature search are currently used in the statistical models of the toolkit. They will be replaced over time by the results of an ongoing systematic review and meta-analysis within the project [21]. However, the used information can get outdated when new corona variants become established and then have to be updated. Currently, the package bundles the statistical models for the several COVID-19 use cases. In the future, further models for other infectious diseases, which have the potential to help the local health authorities in certain situations, could be developed and added to the package.

5. Conclusion

We introduced a decision support application for local health authorities. It contains several tools based on statistical models for different use cases of COVID-19 cases and their contacts. The web application as well as the package smidm including the statistical models are or will available on the internet. The developed web application has the potential to support the daily work of employees at local health authorities. In future work, the usage of our decision support application by employees will be evaluated and the used statistical models will be validated with simulation studies.

Declarations

Acknowledgements: We thank Stefanie Grimm, Peter Schmitz and Amelie Lucker from the Fraunhofer Institute for Industrial Mathematics ITWM and Hajo Zeeb and Sophia Brüssermann from the Leibniz Institute for Preventive Research and Epidemiology BIPS for the fruitful collaboration in the EsteR project.

Conflict of Interest: The authors declare that there is no conflict of interest.

Contributions of the authors: SJ and RA wrote the first version of the manuscript. SJ, RA, LK, JS, BG and MW revised the manuscript. LK, RA and SJ reviewed the literature. SJ and RA developed the statistical models and the web application. MW supervised the research. All authors have approved the manuscript as submitted and accept responsibility for the scientific integrity of the work.

Funding: This work was funded by the German Federal Ministry of Education and Research (BMBF, Project EsteR, Funding Code: 13GW0542).

References

[1] Ullrich A, Schranz M, Rexroth U, Hamouda O, Schaade L, Diercke M, Boender TS, Robert Koch's Infectious Disease Surveillance Group. Impact of the COVID-19 pandemic and associated non-pharmaceutical interventions on other notifiable infectious diseases in Germany: An analysis of national surveillance data during week 1–2016–week 32–2020. The Lancet Regional Health-Europe. 2021; 6: 100103.

[2] Linden M, Dehning J, Mohr SB, Mohring J, Meyer-Hermann M, Pigeot I, Schöbel A, Priesemann V. Case numbers beyond contact tracing capacity are endangering the containment of COVID-19. Deutsches Ärzteblatt International. 2020; 117(46): 790.

[3] Jiang X, Coffee M, Bari A, Wang J, Jiang X, Huang J, Shi J, Dai J, Cai J, Zhang T, Wu Z, He G, Huang Y. Towards an artificial intelligence framework for data-driven prediction of coronavirus clinical severity. Computers, Materials & Continua. 2020; 63(1): 537-551.

[4] van der Schaar M, Alaa AM, Floto A, Gimson A, Scholtes S, Wood A, McKinney E, Jarret D, Lio P, Ercole A. How artificial intelligence and machine learning can help healthcare systems respond to COVID-19. Machine Learning. 2020; 110(1): 1-14.

[5] Mandal M, Jana S, Nandi SK, Khatua A, Adak S, Kar TK. A model based study on the dynamics of COVID-19: Prediction and control. Chaos Solitons Fractals, 2020, 136: 109889.

[6] Maheshwari P, Alber R. Network model and analysis of the spread of Covid-19 with social distancing. Applied Network Science. 2020; 5(100): 1-13.

[7] Bustamante-Casteneda F, Caputo JG, Cruz-Pacheco G, Knippel A, Mouatamide F. Epidemic model on a network: Analysis and applications to COVID-19. Physica A: Statistical Mechanics and its Applications. 2021; 564: 125520.

[8] Lelieveld J, Helleis F, Borrmann S, Cheng Y, Drewnick F, Haug G, Klimach T, Sciare J, Su H, Pöschl U. Model Calculations of Aerosol Transmission and Infection Risk of COVID-19 in Indoor Environments. International Journal of Environmental Research and Public Health. 2020; 17(21): 8114.

[9] The microCOVID Project. 2022 https://www.microcovid.org

[10] Faensen D, Claus H, Benzler J, Ammon A, Pfoch T, Breuer T, Krause G. SurvNet@RKI -- a multistate electronic reporting system for communicable diseases. Euro Surveillance. 2006; 11(4): 7-8.

[11] Tom-Aba D, Silenou BC, Doerrbecker J, Fourie C, Leitner C, Wahnschaffe M, Strysewske M, Arinze CC, Krause G. The Surveillance Outbreak Response Management and Analysis System (SORMAS): Digital Health Global Goods Maturity Assessment JMIR Public Health Surveillance. 2020; 6(2): e15860.

[12] Xin H, Wong JY, Murphy C, Yeung A, Taslim Ali S, Wu P, Cowling BJ. The Incubation Period Distribution of Coronavirus Disease 2019: A Systematic Review and Meta-Analysis. Clinical Infectious Diseases, 2021; 73(12): 2344-2352.

[13] Hyndman RJ, Einbeck J, Wand MP. hdrcde: Highest Density Regions and Conditional Density Estimation. R package version 3.4 2021, https://pkg.robjhyndman.com/hdrcde/.

[14] Zhang J, Litvinova M, Wang W, Wang Y, Deng X, Chen X, Li M, Zheng W, Yi L, Chen X, Wu Q, Liang Y, Xiling W, Yang J, Sun K, Longini IM, Halloran E, Wu P, Cowling BJ, Merler S, Viboud C, Vespignani A, Ajelli M, Yu H. Evolving epidemiology and transmission dynamics of coronavirus disease 2019 outside Hubei province, China: a descriptive and modelling study. The Lancet Infectious Diseases. 2020; 20(7): 793-802.

[15] He X, Lau EHY, Wu P, Deng X, Wang J, Hao X, Lao YC, Wong JY, Guan Y, Tan X, Mo X, Chen Y, Liao B, Chen W, Hu F, Zhang Q, Zhong M, Wi Y, Zhao L, Zhang F, Cowling BJ, Li F, Leung GM. Temporal dynamics in viral shedding and transmissibility of COVID-19. Nature Medicine. 2020; 26: 672–675.

[16] Robert Koch-Institute. Kontaktpersonen-Nachverfolgung (KP-N) bei SARS-CoV-2-Infektionen. https://www.rki.de/DE/Content/InfAZ/N/Neuartiges_Coronavirus/Kontaktperson/Management.html.

[17] Davies NG, Klepac P, Liu Y, Prem K, Jit M, CMMID COVID-19 working group, Eggo RM. Age-dependent effects in the transmission and control of COVID-19 epidemics. Nature Medicine 2020; 26: 1205-1211.

[18] Jäckle S, Röger E, Dicken V, Geisler B, Schumacher J, Westphal M. A Statistical Model to Assess Risk for Supporting COVID-19 Quarantine Decisions. International Journal of Environmental Research and Public Health. 2021; 18(17): 9166.

[19] R Core Team. R: A language and environment for statistical computing. R Foundation for Statistical Computing, 2020, Vienna, Austria. https://www.R-project.org/.

[20] Chang W, Cheng J, Allaire JJ, Sievert C, Schloerke B, Xie Y, Allen J, McPherson J, Dipert A, Borges B. shiny: Web Application Framework for R. R package version 1.6.0. 2021. https://CRAN.R-project.org/package=shiny.

[21] Kühne L, Brüssermann S, De Santis KK, Zeeb H. EsteR – Decision support for German health authorities by risk modelling in order to contain the COVID-19 pandemic. Protocol for a rapid review. OSF Preprints. 2022. https://osf.io/vq64r/

German Medical Data Sciences 2022 - Future Medicine
R. Röhrig et al. (Eds.)
© 2022 The authors and IOS Press.
doi:10.3233/SHTI220800

Machine Learning Based Classification of Depression Using Motor Activity Data and Autoregressive Model

Alexander SCHULTE[a] and Tim BREIKSCH[a] and Jonas BROCKMANN[a] and
Nadja BAUER[a1]

[a] *University of Applied Sciences and Arts Dortmund*

Abstract. Machine learning based disease classification have already achieved amazing results in medicine: for example, models can find a tumor in computer tomography images at least as accurately as experts in the field. Since the development and widespread use of actigraphy watches, activity data has been used as a basis for diagnosing various diseases such as depression or Alzheimer's disease. In this study, we use a dataset with activity measurements of mentally ill and healthy people, calculate various features and achieve a classification accuracy of over 78%. The paper describes and motivates the used features, discusses differences between healthy, bipolar 2 and unipolar participants and compares several well-known machine learning classifiers on different classification tasks and with different feature sets.

Keywords. Machine learning, depression classification, actometer data, actigraphy watch, depresjon dataset, autoregressive model

1. Introduction

Depression is a serious problem and the most common mental illness in the population. The Global Burden of Diseases, Injuries, and Risk Factors Study (GBD) 2019 rank depressive disorders under the top 25 burdens worldwide in 2019 [6]. [3] show that the COVID-19 pandemic noticeably impacts the mental health of the population as the infection rates are associated with increased prevalence of major depressive disorder. Even though there are often no clear physical signs, the illness can have a disruptive effect on the life of an affected person over an indefinite period of time. A distinction can be made between different types and intensities, which can result in quite different progressions of the disease. Bipolar depression is characterized not only by the classic phases of lack of motivation - as common for unipolar depression - but also by opposite, impulsive phases [4]. A correct classification can thus help to assess the possible extent of the depression more precisely and to improve possible treatment.

Richter et al. [10] summarize in their overview study different machine learning (ML) based behavioral diagnostics tools for depression. The authors distinguish between neuroimaging data (such as brain network patterns) and behavioral data, the latter being divided into social media usage and movement sensor data. The behavioral data are

---

[1] Corresponding Author, Dr. Nadja Bauer, Lecturer at the Faculty of Computer Science, University of Applied Sciences and Arts Dortmund, E-mail: nadja.bauer@fh-dortmund.de.

particularly interesting for diagnostic purposes because they are generally easier to obtain. In this paper, we deal with movement sensor data and give a short overview of related works in this subfield.

Berle et al. [1] provide one of the first studies for distinguishing the movement patterns of healthy and mentally ill people. They collect actigraphy watch data over a two-week period from both groups. The used features are activity averages (full-time and nights), as well as interdaily and intradaily stability (measurement of the strength of circadian rhythmicity). The main conclusion is that mentally ill patients tend to show a lower motor activity as well as a more structured behavior than the control group. However, ML techniques for automated disease classification were not applied. Parts of this dataset have been published by [5] for research purposes and form the basis for the analysis in this paper.

Garcia-Ceja et al. [5] have not only published the so-called "depresjon" dataset, but have already applied different ML methods and compared the results. However, the underlying features are not mentioned. Linear SVM was shown to be the best method with an accuracy of 72.7%. The accuracy of the so called zeroR-classifier (assignment of majority class) is 58%. Authors emphasize the need for sophisticated feature engineering.

Currently, many studies are being conducted worldwide in this direction. [8] compare activity data of older (mostly female) single people with (n=18) and without (n=29) depression. Used features include activity averages, light condition and various sleep parameters, showing low levels of daytime activity for depressed individuals in particular. Logistic regression showed by far the best classification accuracy with 91%, random forest reaches 67% and zeroR 61%.

Minaeva et al. [9] analyze two (not freely available) datasets (development and validation) with activity data of depressed patients, looking at a variety of features, including sleep behavior and some parameters of the fitted circadian curve. The development dataset includes 43 depressive and 82 non-depressive people, with a validation set of 27 people for each group. Backward stepwise logistic regression is used as a ML-method. The classification accuracy on the development dataset amounts to 71.8 % (zeroR accuracy: 65.6 %). For the validation dataset, instead of an accuracy only an AUC value is reported, being 0.65. After backward selection two activity data driven features were left: average of daily gross motor activity and acrophase (time of maximum activity levels across 24-hour periods).

Rodríguez-Ruiz et al. [11] also use the "depresjon" dataset and report an almost perfect accuracy of 99%. However, a closer look reveals inaccuracies. The original time series are divided into segments of 60 minutes and 24 features (some based on Fourier transformation) are calculated, resulting in a dataset of 11945 observations. Although the data were divided into training and validation sets, it was not excluded that the data of the same individuals occur in both subsets leading to information leakage and hence almost perfect accuracy.

Zanella-Calzada et al. [13] also use the "depresjon" dataset for detecting depressive episodes, achieving an accuracy of 89% for the classification of depressed vs. healthy subjects. However, their results are not comparable with ours in many respects - for one, they claim to have 5895 subjects (2112 cases / 3783 controls), although the linked dataset contains only 23 unipolar and bipolar depressed patients and 32 healthy participants. Thus, the patient data is probably divided into different sections risking information leakage leading to a too optimistic classification accuracy. On the other hand, they use an out-of-bag estimate as validation strategy, which only resembles cross-validated error rates after many repetitions. Our approach is much broader, since we additionally want to distinguish between the two depression types and extract a much larger and heterogeneous set of features.

Sing et at. [12] follow a very similar procedure as [13]: they divide the original data into a total of 13844 segments with the goal of learning a classification model on these segments. The same features as in [13] are extracted and a random forest model is used as well. The problem of such an approach is that although individual data segments can be well classified into depressed vs. non-depressed ones, it is not possible to make a diagnosis for a person. Indeed, it is quite possible that parts of a person's data segments will be classified as unipolar, another as bipolar 1, and still another as healthy. Therefore, our goal is to classify individuals and not isolated episodes.

2. Data

We use the "depresjon" dataset of [5] mentioned in the introduction. It consists of two groups: the so-called conditional group of 23 patients with a major depressive disorder and the control group with 32 non-depressive contributors. Each study participant wore an actometer for about two weeks. The wrist-mounted actometers recorded any motion above 0.05g with a sampling frequency of 32Hz leading to data entries in minute intervals. 15 patients of the conditional group have a unipolar and 8 a bipolar disorder. However, for bipolar patients there is a distinction between bipolar 1 and bipolar 2 disorders, while there is only one person with a bipolar 1 disorder. Therefore, we excluded the corresponding data, leading to a dataset with 54 participants.

Some datasets contain long episodes of zero data (probably caused by taking off the actigraphy watch) which could negatively influence the results of the machine learning analysis. Hence, if a period of zero data exceeds a certain value, it is removed from the dataset. Starting with smaller values, we concluded that it suffices to focus this filter on the highest occurring periods, using a value of 5760 minutes (corresponding to 4 days), without changing the result in a remarkable way, impacting only four participants from the control group in total (with id numbers 1, 3, 31 and 32).

Although our work relies only on the existing annotated data and compares different ML approaches to classification, it is necessary to question the quality of the data for the generalizability of the results. Only little information is known about the conducted study (see [1]), such as that the control group was composed of hospital employees (n=23) and students (n=5). There are considerably more women in the control group than in the conditional group. Other confounders that could affect the internal and external validity of the study are not discussed. Consequently, the results of papers based on these data should be interpreted with great caution. At the same time, this highlights the need for further data from similar studies that meet a high standard of clinical research to be made freely available to the ML community.

3. Feature Extraction

Since the data are in the format of a time series with over 20 000 samples per person, it is not possible to take each data entry as a feature. Hence, the time series have to be compressed into a small set of meaningful features which then influence the classification accuracy. Some of these features are motivated through state-of-the-art works and others are proposed by the authors. All calculations were conducted in the Java programming language. We will also mention some used package names.

The first batch of features consists of 11 self-explanatory ones that do not require formal definitions: the highest occurring value (*maximum*), as well as the lowest one (*minimum*), the average (*average*), the median (*median*), the mode (*mode*), the standard deviation (*stdDev*), the variance (*variance*), the coefficient of variation (*varCoeff*), the kurtosis (*kurtosis*) over all samples and the number of occurrences of the value 0 (*nullCount*). An additional standard deviation value is calculated based on the average values of each 24-hour interval to check the heterogeneity between days (*dailyDev*). As almost all studies in this area distinguish between day and night activity, we compute the heterogeneity between the averaged night activities (*nightlyDev*), analogue to *dailyDev*, while defining the night as the time from 10 p.m. to 7 a.m. A further sleep quality feature is defined as: *sleepQuality = (1 – (nightlyDev / stdDev))*. The idea is, that individuals with low night activity fluctuations in relation to overall fluctuations will have *sleepQuality* close to 1, while individuals with very similar fluctuation levels overall and during nights will have *sleepQuality* close to 0.

As smoothing is one of the standard tools for time series analysis, the second batch of 5 features is extracted from the smoothed time series after a moving average with a window size of 11 was applied. The following features are then calculated: maximum (*maMax*), minimum (*maMin*), average (*maAverage*), standard deviation (*maStdDev*) and a relative maxima difference defined as: *maxDiffFactor = (max – maMax) / max*. The larger this characteristic is, the more noticeable is the strongest outlier in the time series.

The third batch of 5 features is applied on the Fourier transformed data as this approach was proposed in [11]: maximum (*fftMax*), average (*fftAverage*), standard deviation (*fftStdDev*), variance (*fftVar*), coefficient of variation (*fftVarCoeff*) and kurtosis (*fftKurtosis*). The window size for the Fourier transformation is the length of the respective time series. Calculations were done using the "FFT4J" java package.

Finally, the fourth feature batch is based on an autoregressive (AR) model. The main idea was to investigate whether the behavior of the participants can be predicted well by an ARIMA model as we expect that the "predictability" of the activity patterns could be a good feature to distinguish between control and conditional group (see [1]). An ARIMA model has several parameters: lag order p, degree of differencing d and the order of the moving average q [2]. We tested in first pre-experiments the impact of different parameter settings and have found that the best results can be achieved for p larger than 20, $d=0$ and $q=0$. So, the ARIMA model was reduced to an AR model with $p=25$.

For feature calculations, we first train the AR model on the first two thirds of each person's activity data and then predict the next activity value t_n as well as the lower and upper confidence bounds for the prediction. Then the absolute difference between the true and the predicted value for t_n is calculated. Furthermore, the normalized variance for the prediction (prediction variance divided by variance of the fitted model) and the root mean squared error for the trained model are noted (as a measurement for model uncertainty and goodness of model fit, respectively). In the next successive steps, the training data is extended by t_n and the model is trained once again for predicting t_{n+1}. Finally, the computed features for all prediction steps are averaged resulting in: *arPredError, arLowerConf, arUpperConf, arNormVar, arRootMeanSqrtError*. The Java package "timeseries-forecast" was used for these calculations.

4. Explorative Data Analysis

In this section explorative comparisons of features depending on the group of participants will be provided. Here we divide the conditional group into bipolar and unipolar patients. Fig. 1 compares the activity data (after applying the moving average as described above) of two participants: one from the control group (A) und one from the conditional group (B) for a time period of two weeks. First, clear day-night cycles are visible. The comparison shows a clear difference in average activity: in general, the healthy person seems to be more active than the other one. This behavior is measurable across almost all cases as can be seen in Fig. 2 (a) for the *average* feature. Similar to findings in [1], [8] or [9], higher activity of the control group can also be stated when comparing the features *maximum, stdDev, variance, median, dailyDev* and *mode*.

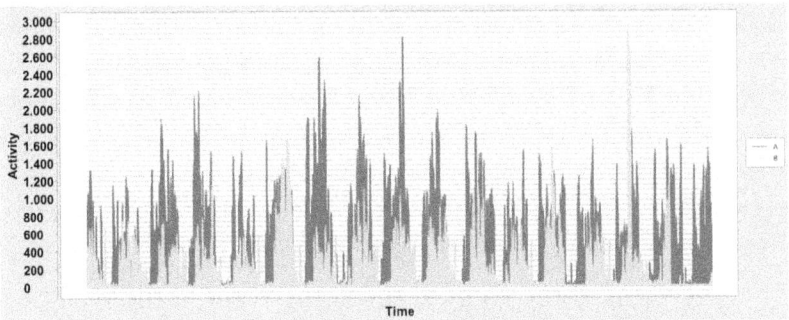

Figure 1. Activity data (after applying moving average) of a healthy participant (A) and of a participant with unipolar depression (B).

The *kurtosis* and *varCoeff* features show no meaningful difference between healthy, bipolar 2 or unipolar individuals. The *minimum* activity of each dataset is 0 and therefore this feature is irrelevant for further classification. The conditional group shows an increased *nullCount* value compared to the control group, which can again be explained by lower activity. The *sleepQuality* of bipolar 2 patients seems to be lower than for other participants (see Fig. 2 (b)). This can be explained with the higher *nightlyDev* of this group.

The moving average batch of features yields similar results: higher values for the *maMax, maAverage* and *maStdDev* features for the control group. Unipolar patients show a higher *maxDiffFactor* value compared to healthy and bipolar 2 participants, which could be an indicator for higher "extreme values" in their activity.

For the frequency domain-based attributes from the third feature batch the following can be stated: the attributes *fftVar, fftStdDev* and *fftMax* have higher values for the healthy control group, while for *fftAverage* and *fftVarCoeff* no clear differences between the groups can be observed. The value of *fftKurtosis* for the conditional group (especially for bipolar 2 patients) is lower compared to the healthy group (see Fig. 2 (d)). Spectral kurtosis is an indicator for randomly occurring fluctuation in the activity profile, so depressive patients seem to me more "predictable" in their activity patterns.

The last batch with AR based features also shows differences between bipolar 2, unipolar and healthy participants. The value for *arPredError* is substantially lower for depressed patients of both kinds compared to healthy participants, although bipolar 2 patients retain a higher value than unipolar patients (see Fig. 2 (d)). Hence, participants with a unipolar disorder seem to have more structured activity patterns. *arRootMeanSquareError* values are in general lower for depressed patients meaning a better model fit for this group. However, the condition group shows higher *arNormVar* values compared to the healthy control group, which might be caused by smaller variances of the fitted models. According to the distribution of the *arLowerConf* and *arUpperConf* features, the bipolar 2 patients show smaller prediction intervals than other participants.

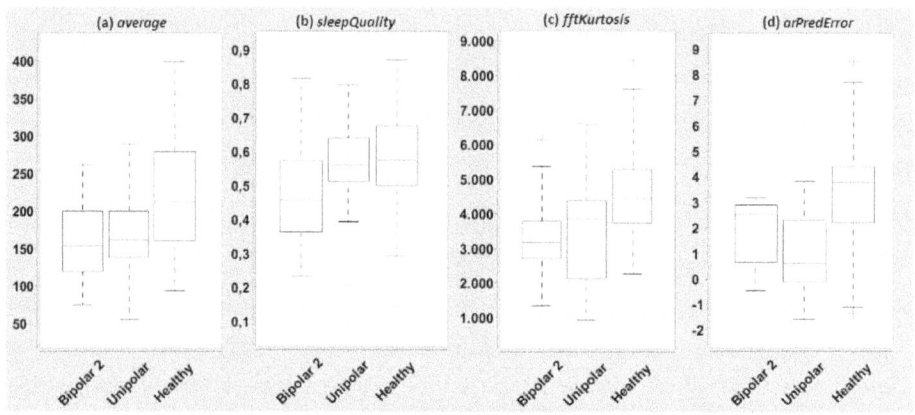

Figure 2. Distribution comparison of some selected features for three groups: patients with bipolar 2 disorder, patients with unipolar disorder and healthy participants (control group).

5. Machine Learning based Classification

The theoretical aspects of machine learning techniques applied in this paper (like classifiers, validation, performance measures) can be found in [7].

The following classification tasks will be considered: 1) unipolar vs. non-unipolar, 2) bipolar 2 vs. non-bipolar 2, 3) healthy vs. non-healthy (bipolar and unipolar) participants. Especially for the second task the problem of unbalanced classes occurs as there are only seven bipolar 2 patients against 47 non-bipolar 2 participants. For this reason, we will compare the classification results with the zeroR-classifier (classification to the majority class). Furthermore, in order to measure the impact of AR based features three sets of features are compared: 1) "No AR" - all features except for the AR batch, 2) "AR only" - only AR based features and 3) "Combined" - all features. We compare RandomForest, AdaBoost and LogReg (logistic regression) classifiers, as these approaches count to the top data mining algorithms and in order to verify the remarkably good performance of logistic regression in [8]. Machine learning was realized using the Java library "Smile".

To avoid overfitting, 50 times replicated 10-fold cross validation is applied and measured by the classification accuracy. As a reminder, the dataset consists of 54 observations, 26 features and a target variable with three labels (unipolar / bipolar 2 / healthy). The results are presented in Table 1, while the best result for each classification task is highlighted in bold. The main finding is that the AR features seem to lead to a relevant improvement of the classification accuracy for all three tasks, while for bipolar 2 vs. non-bipolar 2 and for healthy vs. non-healthy classification "AR only" shows the best results. Logistic regression achieves better results on extremely unbalanced classification tests (bipolar 2 vs non-bipolar 2), slightly beating the zeroR-classifier. AdaBoost performs better on both other tasks with accuracies clearly better than the zeroR-classification.

The achieved accuracies (especially for healthy vs. non-healthy task) seem to outperform the state-of-the-art results. In order to verify the feature importance, we applied RandomForest and AdaBoost models on the whole dataset for the healthy vs. non-healthy classification task and computed variable importance values. The top tree features for RandomForest are: *arPredError*, *fftMax* and *mode*, and for AdaBoost: *average* (by far), *nullCount* and *arPredError*.

Table 1. Results of the classification benchmark. Validation criterion: accuracy measure, validation strategy: 50 times replicated 10-fold cross validation

Classification task	Classifier	Feature set		
		No AR	AR only	Combined
unipolar vs. non-unipolar	RandomForest	74.07 %	74.27 %	76.93 %
	AdaBoost	66.53 %	72.27 %	**79.33 %**
	LogReg	73.85 %	78.71 %	71.90 %
	zeroR	72.22 %	72.22 %	72.22 %
Bipolar 2 vs. non-bipolar 2	RandomForest	87,16 %	87.33 %	87.20 %
	AdaBoost	81,47 %	80.00 %	84.60 %
	LogReg	87.33 %	87.28 %	**87.39 %**
	zeroR	87.04 %	87.04 %	87.04 %
Healthy vs. non-healthy	RandomForest	65.59 %	76.87 %	70.60 %
	AdaBoost	68.30 %	**78.40 %**	75.00 %
	LogReg	59.30 %	76.05 %	59.20 %
	zeroR	59.26 %	59.26 %	59.26 %

6. Discussion

In this paper we compared several state-of-the-art features and models for the ML based detection of unipolar and bipolar 2 depression disorder - the most common psychiatric disorders worldwide. The features based on the prediction ability of an AR model seem to contribute relevant improvements to the classification accuracy leading to better results than in related works (78 % accuracy for heathy vs. non-healthy classification). However, the shortcoming of our study is the small dataset. Our requests regarding further data on several researchers remained unanswered. A larger amount of high-quality data could eventually make it possible to create reliable ML-models with as few features as possible to assist physicians based on a patient's activity patterns alone. Of course, it should be noted that this can only be used in practice once a model is proven by further prospective performance evaluation testing.

7. Declarations

Conflict of Interest: The authors declare that there is no conflict of interest.

Author contributions: AS, TB, JB: conception of the work, conduction of experiments and first draft of the manuscript; NB: mentoring, substantial revision of the manuscript.

References

[1]   Berle JO, Hauge ER, Oedegaard KJ, Holsten F, Fasmer OB. Actigraphic registration of motor activity reveals a more structured behavioural pattern in schizophrenia than in major depression. BMC Res Notes. 2010 May 27;3:149.

[2]   Box E P, Jenkins, GM. Time series analysis: Forecasting and control. San Francisco: Holden-Day; 1970.

[3]   COVID-19 Mental Disorders Collaborators. Global prevalence and burden of depressive and anxiety disorders in 204 countries and territories in 2020 due to the COVID-19 pandemic. Lancet. 2021 Nov 6;398(10312):1700-1712.

[4]   Cuellar AK, Johnson SL, Winters R. Distinctions between bipolar and unipolar depression. Clin Psychol Rev. 2005 May;25(3):307-39.

[5]   Garcia-Ceja E, Riegler M, Jakobsen P, Tørresen J, Nordgreen T, Oedegaard KJ, Fasmer OB. Depresjon: A Motor Activity Database of Depression Episodes in Unipolar and Bipolar Patients, In MMSys'18 Proceedings of the 9th ACM on Multimedia Systems Conference, Amsterdam, The Netherlands, 2018 June; 12-15.

[6]   GBD 2019 Diseases and Injuries Collaborators. Global burden of 369 diseases and injuries in 204 countries and territories, 1990-2019: a systematic analysis for the Global Burden of Disease Study 2019. Lancet. 2020 Oct 17;396(10258):1204-1222.

[7]   Hastie, T, Tibshirani R, Friedman, J. The elements of statistical learning: data mining, inference and prediction. Springer; 2009.

[8]   Kim H, Lee S, Lee S, Hong S, Kang H, Kim N. Depression Prediction by Using Ecological Momentary Assessment, Actiwatch Data, and Machine Learning: Observational Study on Older Adults Living AloneJMIR Mhealth Uhealth 2019;7(10).

[9]   Minaeva O, Riese H, Lamers F, Antypa N, Wichers M, Booij SH. Screening for Depression in Daily Life: Development and External Validation of a Prediction Model Based on Actigraphy and Experience Sampling Method. J Med Internet Res. 2020 Dec 1;22(12).

[10] Richter T, Fishbain B, Richter-Levin G, Okon-Singer H. Machine Learning-Based Behavioral Diagnostic Tools for Depression: Advances, Challenges, and Future Directions. J Pers Med. 2021 Sep 26;11(10):957.

[11] Rodríguez-Ruiz JG, Galván-Tejada CE, Vázquez-Reyes S, Galván-Tejada JI, Gamboa-Rosales H. Classification of Depressive Episodes Using Nighttime Data; a Multivariate and Univariate Analysis. Programming and Computer Software; Dec 2020; 46(8): 689-698.

[12] Singh PM, Sathidevi PS. (2022). Design and Implementation of a Machine Learning-Based Technique to Detect Unipolar and Bipolar Depression Using Motor Activity Data. In Smart Trends in Computing and Communications. 2022; 99-107. Springer Singapore.

[13] Zanella-Calzada LA, Galván-Tejada CE, Chávez-Lamas NM, Gracia-Cortés M, Magallanes-Quintanar R, Celaya-Padilla JM, Galván-Tejada JI, Gamboa-Rosales H. Feature extraction in motor activity signal: Towards a depression episodes detection in unipolar and bipolar patients. Diagnostics. 2019; 9(1): 8.

German Medical Data Sciences 2022 - Future Medicine
R. Röhrig et al. (Eds.)

doi:10.3233/SHTI220801

Consistency of Feature Importance Algorithms for Interpretable EEG Abnormality Detection

Felix KNISPEL[a], Alexander BRENNER[b], Rainer RÖHRIG[a], Yvonne WEBER[c],
Julian VARGHESE[b], and Ekaterina KUTAFINA[a,d,1]

[a] Institute of Medical Informatics, Medical Faculty, RWTH Aachen University, Aachen,
Germany
[b] Institute of Medical Informatics, University of Münster, Münster, Germany
[c] Department of Epileptology, Neurology, Medical Faculty, RWTH Aachen University,
Aachen, Germany
[d] Faculty of Applied Mathematics, AGH University of Science and Technology,
Krakow, Poland

Abstract. Recent advances in machine learning show great potential for automatic detection of abnormalities in electroencephalography (EEG). While simple and interpretable models combined with expert-comprehensible input features offer full control of the decision making process, these methods commonly lag behind complex deep learning and feature extraction methods in terms of performance. Here we study a feasibility of a bridging solution, where deep learning is combined with interpretable input and an algorithm computing the importance of particular EEG features in the decision process. We built a convolutional neural network with multi-channel EEG frequency bands as input and investigated four different methods for feature importance attribution: Layer-wise Relevance Propagation (LRP), DeepLIFT, Integrated Gradients (IG) and Guided GradCAM. Our analysis showed consistency between the first three methods, and deviating attributions of the fourth method, suggesting the importance of using a package of methods together to ensure the robustness of medical interpretation.

Keywords. Machine Learning Interpretability, Electroencephalography, EEG, Decision Support Techniques

1. Introduction

Modern machine learning (ML) systems are increasingly considered as an important tool in clinical decision support systems. However, some domains, such as electroencephalography (EEG) that measures electrical brain activity, remain challenging. An important issue remains the lack of transparency and interpretability of the best performing models, which typically use raw data or highly complex features as an input to the black box of deep learning neural networks.

---

[1] Corresponding Author: Dr. Ekaterina Kutafina, PhD. Address: Institute of Medical Informatics, Medical Faculty, RWTH Aachen University, Pauwelsstraße 30, 52074 Aachen, Germany. Email: ekutafina@ukaachen.de

In [1] we constructed an ML model to detect abnormalities in EEG recordings on the example of the Temple University Hospital (TUH) dataset [2]. In [3] we worked towards an understanding of the individual computational steps that lead to a classification of an EEG. The importance of individual EEG channels and the generated features in general was analyzed. Another possible direction of improvement is combining expert-interpretable features with deep learning models. In such setup, post hoc interpretability algorithms can be used to determine the importance of a given feature in the decision process. As a result, explanations of model decisions can be given in a user-interpretable format. In this paper, we explored this direction by building up on our previous work. We replaced difficult to comprehend wavelet input features with clinically-relevant frequency bands. These features were mapped to a grid for all electrode positions, generating an approximate head-map per sample. The resulting images were used as input to a deep learning (DL) model. This approach allowed us to consider different post hoc feature attribution methods and discuss their consistency and possible relationship with the results to the medical reasoning.

The choice of the feature attribution methods is based on several works published on EEG interpretability. The Layer-Wise Relevance Propagation (LRP) has been previously applied to BCI-EEG data in [4] to generate heatmaps of feature importance. This way, Sturm and colleagues were able to explain with high-resolution at what point in time and at which electrodes on the head scalp the electrical activity was important in the model's classification. Uyttenhove et al. [5] applied a different feature attribution method, GradCAM, to raw time-series EEG data to obtain clinically plausible attributions. DeepLIFT was used by Jansen et al. [6] to analyze the results of an artificial neural network trained on physiological network data of insomnia patients. Integrated Gradients (IG) is another common method for highlighting feature attributions [7].

2. Methods

MNE (v0.24.1) [8] was used for accessing EEG data. PyTorch (v1.10.1) was used to develop and evaluate the machine learning model. To generate feature attributions using LRP, GradCAM, DeepLIFT and IG, we used Captum (v0.4.1) [9].

2.1. Data

The openly available Temple University Hospital (TUH) Abnormal EEG Corpus v2.0.0 [2] is used as our example. 2993 EEG sessions from 2383 subjects are included. Of those sessions, 93% were recorded with a sampling frequency of 250 Hz, the remaining sessions were sampled with 256 or 512 Hz. 1472 recordings are labeled as abnormal, the remaining 1521 as normal. The labeling of EEGs by the dataset authors is based on visual analysis of frequency, voltage, waveform, regulation, locus, reactivity and interhemispheric coherence [2]. The recordings are split into a training set of 2717 recordings and an evaluation set consisting of 276 recordings. We trained models exclusively on the training set, and report model accuracy and feature attributions on the evaluation set.

2.2. Preprocessing

Similar to Brenner et al. [1] and Mortaga et al. [3], we extracted the first minute of every EEG recording. All 21 electrodes were used. The 60 seconds of raw data were re-sampled to 250 Hz, band-filtered (1-50 Hz), and then divided into 11 sliding windows, each of 10 second length with a 5 second overlap. Each segment was checked against a threshold for maximal amplitude. If more than 50% of all electrodes exceeded this threshold, the segment was removed. Lastly, on each remaining segment we calculated power spectral density (PSD) for the five clinically relevant frequency ranges (Delta: 1-3 Hz, Theta: 4-7 Hz, Alpha: 8-13 Hz, Beta: 14-30 Hz, Gamma: >30 Hz) using Welch's method with Hann windowing and 50% overlap. Our final dataset consisted of 27761 segments in the training set and 2813 segments in the testing set, with 5 PSD values for every single one of the 21 electrodes. Each segment was transformed into a 5x5x7 matrix that can be interpreted as a 5x7 image with five channels corresponding to the five frequency bands. All 21 electrodes were mapped as illustrated on Figure 1 – positions in the matrix without annotated electrodes were assigned zero-values to fill up the matrix format. These "images" consisting out of 175 individual features were used as input to the DL model.

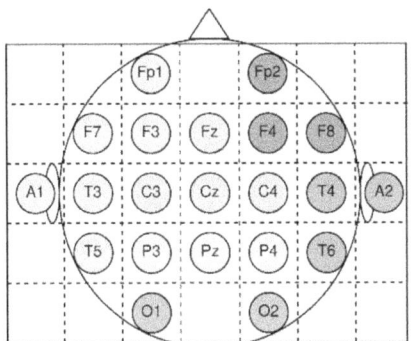

Figure 1. Grid used for mapping electrode positions into a 2D square. The colors illustrate the grouping per brain region used in algorithm comparison.

2.3. Deep Learning model

We constructed a Convolutional Neural Network (CNN) model to classify our segments as normal or abnormal. Our model consists of one convolutional layer (with 3x3 filters), a pooling layer, one fully connected layer with 128 nodes and a final output layer with two nodes representing the class probabilities. Due to the splitting of each EEG recording into 11 segments, we hypothesize that not all segments of an abnormal EEG exhibit abnormal morphologies. This may result in a decreased classification accuracy, as possibly normal-looking segments are labeled as abnormal. To mitigate this problem, we implemented a voting mechanism as in [1].

2.4. Post hoc feature importance attribution

To understand and interpret the importance of our input features, we generated feature importance values using LRP [4], Guided GradCAM [5], DeepLIFT [6], and IG [7] for all 2813 testing segments. Note, that for GradCAM, we obtain relevance scores for the first convolutional layer. These algorithms make use of the given sample, network structure, learned network weights, as well as outcome class of interest. For each of the 175 individual input features, the algorithms return a (positive or negative) real number, indicating an importance of this feature to the outcome of interest. Positive attributions for a feature indicate that high feature values contribute towards the outcome of interest, while negative attributions indicate that low feature values contribute to the outcome of interest. Large absolute feature attributions are therefore considered important features. As our primary interest lies in the reasoning for why an EEG is considered abnormal by the model, we attributed feature importance for the abnormal class.

2.5. Normalization and comparison of feature importance attribution

Due to varying distribution and scale of different feature attribution methods, we applied the following normalization. Outlier removal was performed by first calculating the sum of all attributions for each segment and method. Based on the top and bottom third percentile of attributions for each method, we removed outlier segments. Following this, we normalized every attribution left across electrodes and channels to unit norm using L2-normalization before further processing the attributions.

To view feature importance not only per sample but also across the evaluation set, we averaged attributions for abnormality across all samples. Further, we grouped electrodes into lobes (Frontal left: Fp1, F3, F7; Frontal right: Fp2, F4, F8; Temporal left: A1, T3, T5; Temporal right: A2, T4, T6; Parietal: P3, Pz, P4; Occipital: O1, O2; Central: Fz, Cz, C3, C4). To compare similarity between different methods, we calculated Mean Squared Error (MSE). For every combination of two feature attribution methods, we calculated MSE in attribution differences of a fixed feature (pairing of electrode and frequency band) for every single sample. We then averaged resulting MSE across all features, resulting in one MSE-based score for every combination of methods.

3. Results

During preprocessing, around 7% of all EEG segments were removed due to amplitude thresholding. After training the model, we achieved an accuracy of around 78% on the 2813 segments of the testing set. When using the voting mechanism, accuracy increases to 81.4%. Model performance remains within acceptable range for the study purpose on the test set. This is on par with previous results of 80.15% accuracy in [3], outperforms the results of de Diego [2] (78.8%), but lags behind more complex models such as BD-Deep4 (85.4%) [10] or ChronoNet (86.6%) [11]. Feature attributions were calculated for all test segments using all four methods. After removing 445 of these segments due to outlier values, we normalized and plotted results in Figure 2 and Figure 3. They visualize the attributions generated by the four methods for different electrodes/lobes and frequency bands.

Results of the MSE-based similarity between methods are presented in Figure 4. A single MSE value is difficult to interpret, but Figure 4 shows high agreement between the results of LRP, IG, and DeepLIFT compared to agreement between GradCAM and any other method. Similar conclusion can be drawn from Figures 2 and 3.

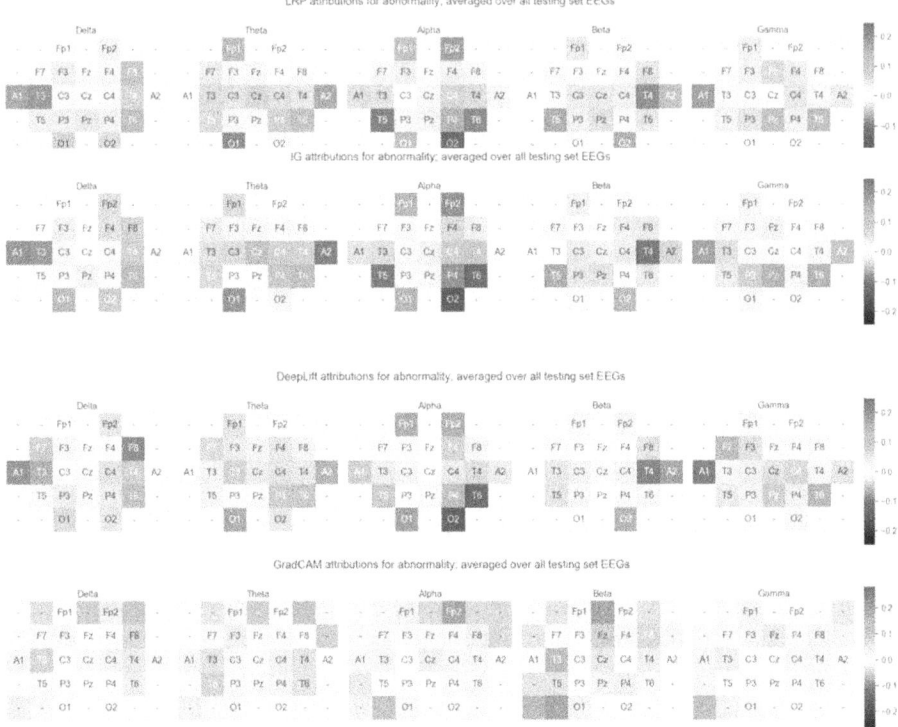

Figure 2. Attributions for abnormality generated by the feature attribution methods.

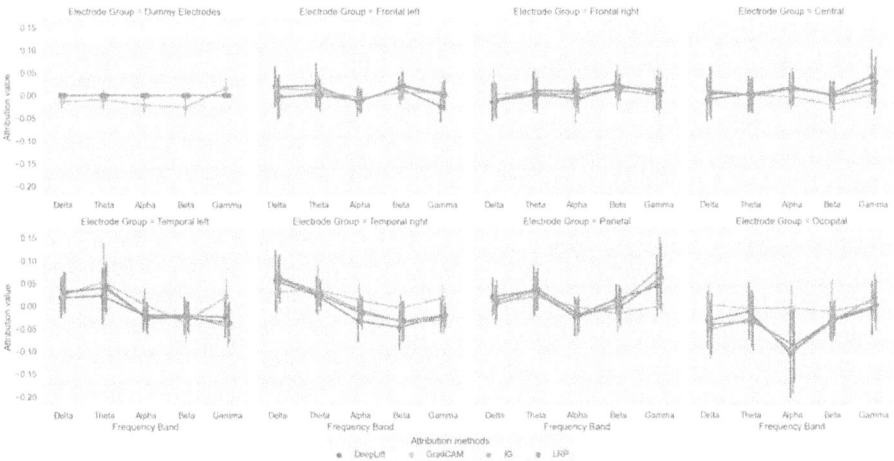

Figure 3. Average attribution values for abnormality, broken down into lobes, methods and frequency bands.

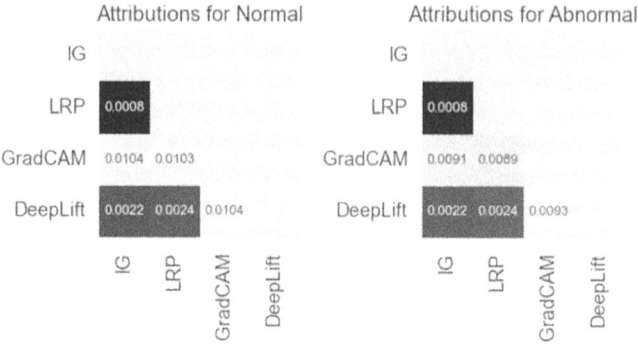

Figure 4. Pairwise mean squared error (MSE) between different attribution methods. Lower MSE indicates higher level of agreement between two methods.

4. Discussion

For the purpose of this study, we have constructed a DL model that uses interpretable frequency-based features extracted from the raw EEG data. The usage of a CNN preserves information about spatial position of the electrodes. As a main paper goal, four different methods for post hoc feature importance assessment were compared by a) using the medically relevant view of the electrode mesh on the head, b) grouping electrodes into larger brain regions and presenting averaged importance attributions separated by frequency bands and brain region and c) computing easy-to-compare MSE.

While our model's performance is notably similar to that of some other models from literature, we note that inferior performance compared to more complex models such as ChronoNet could possibly be attributed to our comparatively simple feature presentation as well as smaller network size.

The head view shows clear visual similarities between three methods with GradCAM being an exception. This is further confirmed by the MSE table (Figure 4) and Figure 3 (line plot). In Figure 2, we can also observe that, in agreement with the expectations, "dummy" electrodes on the 2D grid show little importance. We hypothesize that GradCAM's non-zero feature attribution for these electrodes can be traced back to the method's unique usage of convolutional filters and its handling of Rectified Linear Units in the neural network. Frontal lobes and the central part of the head in general have slightly higher importance. Signals from two temporal lobes (similar directions), parietal (directions opposite to the temporal lobes) and occipital have the strongest effects on the model prediction. High and low frequency bands are showing consistent effects. Interestingly, in the occipital lobe the alpha band clearly stands out, which is in agreement with the fact that large alpha band fluctuation related to e.g. closed/open eyes conditions manifest in the occipital lobe. The medical interpretation of the results should be taken with cautiousness, due to the fact that the labeling of the discussed data set is not controlling for drug usage and it has been reported that medications used to treat epilepsy can affect certain frequency bands [12].

Our work clearly demonstrates both benefits and risks of using feature attribution methods to explain model decisions. On the one hand, calculated feature attributions confirm that the model puts relevance on properties of the EEG signal that are in line with medical expectations. The consistency of some methods allows us to place a certain trust in the functioning of the respective feature attribution methods. On the other hand, inconsistency of others highlights the need for extensive testing and comparison of multiple feature attribution algorithms in the context of EEG data.

In the further work, we will work towards preparing a small data set where both labeled normal and abnormal fragments will be available from the patients who are in an ongoing diagnostic process and therefore are not yet receiving pharmacological intervention. The control for alertness level and age is equally important, as those factors are known to affect the EEG spectrum strongly. Meanwhile, analysis of text-files provided in the TUH dataset for every EEG, describing patient and recording, will be performed. This could enable meaningful validation of feature attributions on the level of individual EEG recordings. Moreover, other datasets in the TUH Corpus contain labels for specific types of abnormalities in EEG recordings. These may be used to further validate obtained results.

5. Conclusion

The paper presents one of several possibilities of constructing human-interpretable ML models for EEG data. The constructed ML model establishes reasonable accuracy, is light weighted and allows to easily test different algorithms for post hoc feature importance attribution. Three of the four tested algorithms showed very consistent results. The inconsistency of the fourth one suggests that if the proposed approach is used for clinical purposes, several different algorithms should be tested to increase the robustness of the importance interpretation.

Declarations

Conflict of Interest: The authors declare that there is no conflict of interest.

Author contributions: FK and AB executed the computations; EK, JV and RR supervised computational side of the work; YW supervised the medical side; FK, EK and AB drafted the manuscript. All authors approved the manuscript in the submitted version and take responsibility for the scientific integrity of the work.

References

[1] Brenner A, Kutafina E, Jonas SM. Automatic recognition of epileptiform EEG abnormalities. In: Building Continents of Knowledge in Oceans of Data: The Future of Co-Created eHealth. IOS Press; 2018. p.171-5.
[2] de Diego, S L. Automated interpretation of abnormal adult electroencephalograms. Temple University. 2017.
[3] Mortaga M, Brenner A, Kutafina E. Towards interpretable machine learning in EEG analysis. In: German Medical Data Sciences 2021: Digital Medicine: Recognize–Understand–Heal. IOS Press; 2021. p. 32-8.
[4] Sturm I, Lapuschkin S, Samek W, Müller KR. Interpretable deep neural networks for single-trial EEG classification. Journal of neuroscience methods. 2016;274:141-5.
[5] Uyttenhove T, Maes A, Van Steenkiste T, Deschrijver D, Dhaene T. Interpretable epilepsy detection in routine, interictal eeg data using deep learning. In: Machine Learning for Health. PMLR; 2020. p. 355-66.

[6]   Jansen C, Penzel T, Hodel S, Breuer S, Spott M, Krefting D. Network physiology in insomnia patients: Assessment of relevant changes in network topology with interpretable machine learning models. Chaos: An Interdisciplinary Journal of Nonlinear Science. 2019;29(12):123129.

[7]   Sundararajan M, Taly A, Yan Q. Axiomatic attribution for deep networks. In: International conference on machine learning. PMLR; 2017. p. 3319-28.

[8]   Gramfort A, Luessi M, Larson E, Engemann DA, Strohmeier D, Brodbeck C, et al. MEG and EEG data analysis with MNE-Python. Frontiers in neuroscience. 2013:267.

[9]   Kokhlikyan N, Miglani V, Martin M, Wang E, Alsallakh B, Reynolds J, et al. Captum: A unified and generic model interpretability library for PyTorch; 2020.

[10]   Tibor Schirrmeister R, Gemein L, Eggensperger K, Hutter F, Ball T. Deep learning with convolutional neural networks for decoding and visualization of eeg pathology. arXiv e-prints. 2017:arXiv-1708.

[11]   Roy S, Kiral-Kornek I, Harrer S. ChronoNet: a deep recurrent neural network for abnormal EEG identification. In: Conference on artificial intelligence in medicine in Europe. Springer; 2019. p. 47-56.

[12]   Ouyang CS, Chiang CT, Yang RC, Wu RC, Wu HC, Lin LC. Quantitative EEG findings and response to treatment with antiepileptic medications in children with epilepsy. Brain and Development.

German Medical Data Sciences 2022 - Future Medicine
R. Röhrig et al. (Eds.)
doi:10.3233/SHTI220802

Secure Multi-Party Computation Based Distributed Feasibility Queries – A HiGHmed Use Case

Reto WETTSTEIN[a,1,2], Tobias KUSSEL[b,2], Hauke HUND[c], Christian FEGELER[c],
Martin DUGAS[a], and Kay HAMACHER[b]

[a]*Institute of Medical Informatics, Heidelberg University Hospital,
Heidelberg, Germany*
[b]*Computational Biology & Simulation, Technical University Darmstadt,
Darmstadt, Germany*
[c]*GECKO Institute, Heilbronn University of Applied Sciences,
Heilbronn, Germany*

Abstract. The integration of routine medical care data into research endeavors promises great value. However, access to this extra-domain data is constrained by numerous technical and legal requirements. The German Medical Informatics Initiative (MII) – initiated by the Federal Ministry of Research and Education (BMBF) – is making progress in setting up Medical Data Integration Centers to consolidate data stored in clinical primary information systems. Unfortunately, for many research questions cross-organizational data sources are required, as one organization's data is insufficient, especially in rare disease research. A first step, for research projects exploring possible multi-centric study designs, is to perform a feasibility query, i.e., a cohort size calculation transcending organizational boundaries. Existing solutions for this problem, like the previously introduced feasibility process for the MII's HiGHmed consortium, perform well for most use cases. However, there exist use cases where neither centralized data repositories, nor Trusted Third Parties are acceptable for data aggregation. Based on open standards, such as BPMN 2.0 and HL7 FHIR R4, as well as the cryptographic techniques of secure Multi-Party Computation, we introduce a fully automated, decentral feasibility query process without any central component or Trusted Third Party. The open source implementation of the proposed solution is intended as a plugin process to the HiGHmed Data Sharing Framework. The process's concept and underlying algorithms can also be used independently.

Keywords. Feasibility queries, distributed processes, privacy, secure multi-party computation, medical informatics, BPMN, FHIR

---

[1] Corresponding Author, Reto Wettstein, Institute of Medical Informatics, Heidelberg University Hospital, Im Neuenheimer Feld 130.3, 69120 Heidelberg, Germany; E-mail: reto.wettstein@med.uni-heidelberg.de

[2] These authors contributed equally

1. Introduction

1.1. Background

The era of big data promises vast advancements in nearly all research fields, be it chronic disease management [1], personalized medicine [2], psychiatry [3], or intensive care research [4]. One way to incorporate this paradigm into medical research is to unlock the use of routine medical care data for research purposes [5]. For this reason, the Medical Informatics Initiative (MII) [6] was established by the German Federal Ministry of Education and Research, aiming to connect Germany's university hospitals with research institutes and health-care businesses. The initiative's primary goal is the development of suitable infrastructures and processes to meet the paradigm. The involved university hospitals are establishing so-called Medical Data Integration Centers (MeDICs), in which data from primary medical information systems' are integrated into research repositories using open standards as well as harmonized interfaces and processes [7,8].

The MII's infrastructure tries to aid medical researchers in many steps of the research process. This work is especially concerned with the step of feasibility queries, a preparatory step for clinical studies in order to determine the size of an available cohort. Many research projects require cohort sizes only achievable by consolidating data of multiple organizations. Unfortunately, even if no identifying patient data are processed, disclosure of aggregated data can still become a privacy risk. Especially for studies dealing with rare diseases, the geographical data of organizations can be used for re-identification, due to the very small number of patients treated at each hospital. Hence, a distributed, privacy-preserving feasibility process based on the cryptographic techniques of secure Multi-Party Computation (MPC) is designed, implemented, and tested.

1.2. Objective and Requirements

The MII Taskforce for Process Modeling, on behalf of the National Steering Committee (NSG), developed a high-level process template describing feasibility queries [9]. Additionally, the MII Data Protection Concept (DSK) [10] describes the legal requirements and gives concrete recommendations. Based on these two documents, a fully decentralized process for feasibility queries in small cohort sizes was developed to meet the more specific requirements of the MII's HiGHmed [11] consortium. These requirements are:

1. An automated, fully decentral process should be employed.
2. Patients' sensitive data must be protected with highest privacy guarantees.
3. The privacy of very small (local) cohort sizes should be protected, no Trusted Third Party (TTP) must be used.
4. The process must be deployable on the HiGHmed framework for data sharing.
5. Interoperability should be ensured by using open standards and data models.

To meet these requirements, the process presented in this work was designed and implemented as a deployable plugin for the HiGHmed Data Sharing Framework (DSF) [12]. It was tested using sample data across three MeDIC organizations. The important steps of this process, the sharing and aggregation of distributed cohort sizes, utilize secure Multi-Party Computation techniques in order to render a TTP superfluous.

2. State of the art

As the task of distributed feasibility queries is a common and necessary step in many medical research endeavors, various platforms that address this question exist. For example, the Clinical Communication Platform implemented by the German Cancer Consortium (DKTK) provides a central search function to request case numbers across the members' patient databases [13]. These requests await approval by the local use and access committees and are released via locally deployed software components. The results, however, disclose the number of patients on an organizational level.

The German Centre for Cardiovascular Research (DZHK) operates an architecture with an orthogonal approach by their Clinical Research Platform, providing a searchable central data repository [14].

In MII's Collaboration on Rare Diseases (CORD-MI) the MPC based analysis tool EasySMPC[3] was developed, aiming for a no-code solution. Its GUI driven usage is well suited for physician-led one-off analyses, however, its application for pipeline integration is limited.

One recent solution, able to meet most requirements, is the HiGHmed Data Sharing Framework (DSF) [12]. It uses a decentralized task queueing system and a process engine based on the open standards HL7 Fast Healthcare Interoperability Resources (HL7 FHIR R4)[4] and Business Process Model and Notation (BPMN 2.0)[5]. These components are deployed at every participating organization – the HL7 FHIR Endpoint as a publicly reachable authentication, authorization, and task queueing system and the Business Process Engine (BPE) in the internal network to execute the requested processes and communicate with local services, e.g., patient data repositories, master patient indices, or consent management services. The existing HiGHmed feasibility process [15] allows decentralized feasibility queries with optional consent checking and optional record linkage. It uses a TTP for data aggregation and record linkage purposes. A similar system, based on the HiGHmed DSF as well, is employed in the network for clinical medicine's (NUM) Covid-19 project CODEX [16].

While the DSF based solutions fulfil most of the given requirements, all of them fail to provide a high level of privacy protection for small local cohort sizes, by requiring a TTP, which might be dealing with few patient data posing a re-identification risk.

In this work, we develop, implement, and test a distributed process for the HiGHmed DSF which enables researchers to perform feasibility queries without a TTP, hence increasing both the privacy level for small local cohort sizes and the overall privacy level by utilizing mathematically provable cryptographic techniques for data protection.

3. Concept

Andrew C. Yao's seminal work [17] started the field of MPC in 1986. It was considered a theoretical technique, until the introduction of the "Fairplay" compiler [18] in 2004 and advancements in computing hardware and protocol optimizations allowed practical applications. Since then, MPC is an active research field, enabling an ever-increasing number of use cases to perform computations over distributed data sets in a privacy-

---

[3] https://github.com/prasser/easy-smpc
[4] https://www.hl7.org/fhir/R4
[5] https://www.omg.org/spec/BPMN/2.0

preserving manner. In principle, every calculation that is achievable using a TTP is achievable *without* a TTP using MPC protocols. However, the performance of MPC protocols is often multiple orders of magnitude slower than plain text analyses. The process is based on an extension of the GMW protocol [19] (named after its authors Goldreich, Micali, and Wigderson) to algebraic rings in order to calculate the total cohort size. Both variants work on secret shares, i.e., the secret input data is "broken up" into two or more parts. These shares do not contain any information in themself. To reconstruct the secret value, *all* shares must be recombined. Even with only one share missing no recombination is possible. By representing the computation functionality as an Arithmetic Circuit consisting of additions and multiplications, any (bounded) computation can be performed.

As feasibility queries only require the addition of values, we can exploit the additive homomorphic property of the arithmetic shares to design a comparatively simple communication protocol, suitable for the implementation into the task- and business process based DSF. The usual bottleneck in MPC performance, the available network bandwidth, does not pose a restriction for feasibility queries, as only small messages need to be transmitted.

Figure 1 illustrates the BPMN model, developed for this task. The topmost pool represents the coordinating organization, the two other pools show subprocesses executed at every participating organization. The final cohort size is calculated in an interactive protocol, the arithmetic shares are reconstructed at the coordinating organization, thus revealing the result. The complete TTP-less feasibility query process consists of the following steps:

First, a researcher defines his feasibility query at the leading organization by providing inclusion and exclusion criteria for cohort size calculation as well as whether consent checking should be performed. Currently the targets of the feasibility query process include all organizations belonging to a consortium in order to mitigate the attack scenario of disclosing individual organizations cohort sizes by performing successive feasibility queries, differing in only one excluded organization.

After the feasibility query has been created, two requests are sent to each participating organization, starting two different subprocesses. Note that both subprocesses, the lower two pools in Figure 1, are logically sequential, dividing the feasibility query execution in two stages. However, to handle network latencies and other artifacts in distributed, concurrent executions, two simultaneously executed subprocesses are involved with one waiting for the results of the other.

The logical first stage consists of the subprocess displayed in the lowest pool. After various validity checks against local and global constraints, the feasibility query is executed. If the researcher indicated to perform consent checking, the query is modified before execution to collect the Patient Identifier (PID) for each queried patient. These PIDs are used, to query the local Policy Decision Point (PDP), whether access to the patient's data has been restricted. Both cases, consent checking or not, result in the local cohort size, which is then *secret shared* (as explained above). For each participating organization one share is generated. One is held locally, the others are transmitted to all other organization, initiating the second stage, illustrated in the middle pool. Note that by withholding one share, no other participating organization can extract any information from the received shares.

In the second stage, all participating organizations wait to receive the respective shares from all other participants. If one or more organization fails to send their share, the process times out and terminates, as there is no possibility to maintain computational

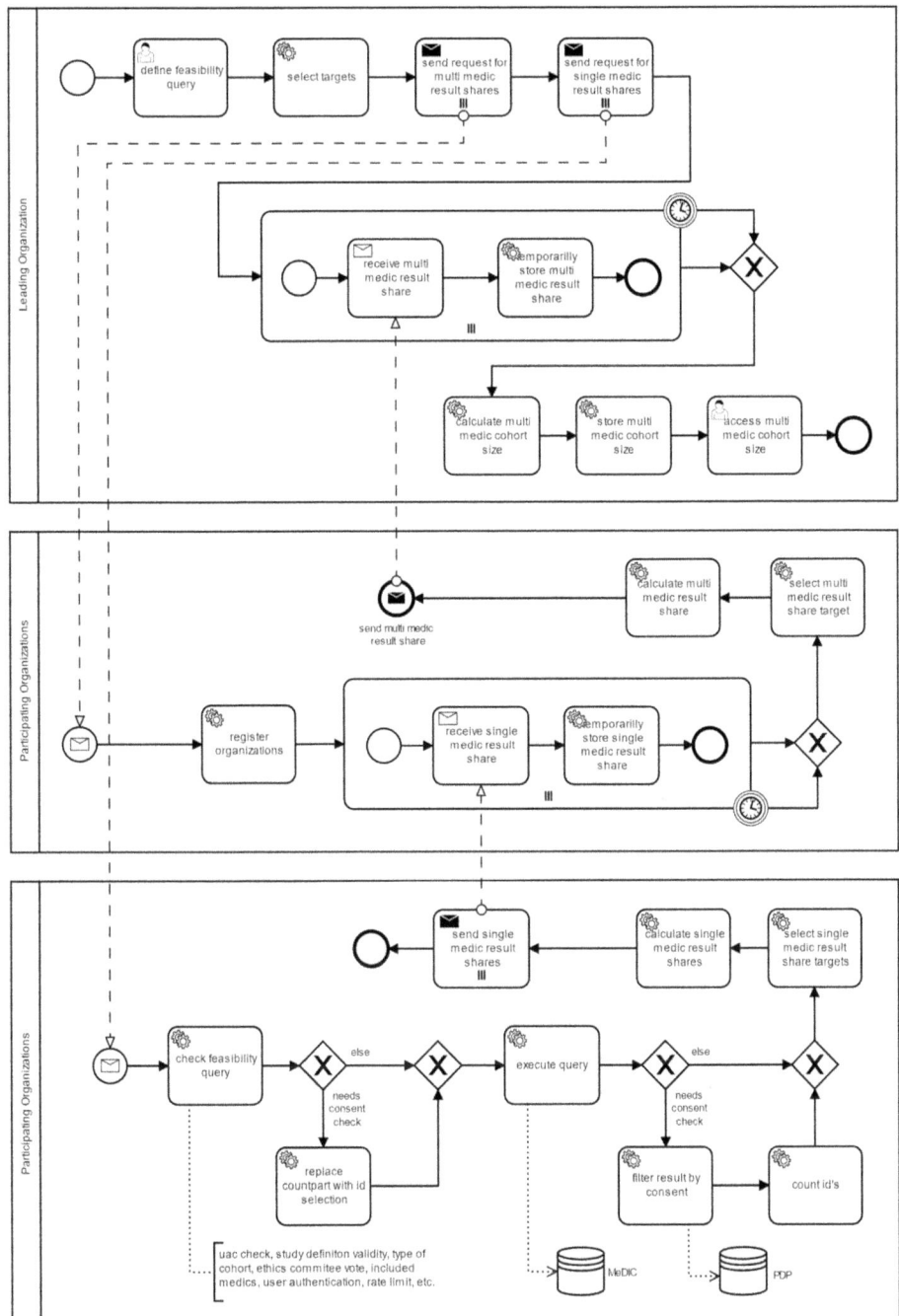

Figure 1. BPMN process diagram of the MPC feasibility process with optional consent checking

correctness with incomplete sets of shares. After all shares have been received, each organization combines the received shares, including their own, withheld one. This combination uses the homomorphic properties of the secret shares: adding all up and performing a modulo operation with the size of the used arithmetic ring, generating a valid secret share of the sum, i.e., of the desired total cohort size. This multi-MeDIC result share is sent to the leading organization, ending the computation.

In the last step, the leading organization awaits the multi-MeDIC result shares from all participating organizations. Upon receiving all of them, the shares can be recombined to reveal the clear text result, the total cohort size. The computation itself is secure against malicious adversaries, i.e., corrupted parties can only prohibit the correct calculation of the result (by injecting wrong input data or failing to send their shares), but not gain any information regarding the other parties' inputs.

4. Implementation

The proposed MPC feasibility process was implemented as a plugin process for the HiGHmed DSF in the Java programming language, using HL7 FHIR R4 resources as data model as well as BPMN 2.0 as process model, in order to remain agnostic of an organization's data repository choices and to establish semantic interoperability. The data and process model specific implementations, such as the profiled FHIR resources ResearchStudy, Group and Task, do not differ from those used in the feasibility process using a TTP for data aggregation [15]. Therefore, we would like to refer the interested reader to [15] for detailed explanations and focus on the employed cryptographic primitives and protocols in the following paragraphs.

For the secret sharing scheme, we chose a ring size of $r = 2^{32} - 1$ to fit all shares in a 32-bit integer type. As we expect cross-organizational cohort sizes of less than around 4.3 billion for virtually all use cases, this size is sufficient. However, a variant using Java's BigInteger data type is implemented, allowing arbitrary ring sizes and values. Each party in a computation with n participants generates n shares by sampling $n - 1$ uniformly independent and identically distributed Integers: $s_i \leftarrow_\$ \{0,1,2,...,$ $2^{32} - 1\}$. The last share is generated by mixing the secret value v with all previously (randomly) generated shares, such that $v = \sum_i s_i \mod r \; \forall i$. Due to the modular arithmetic on the algebraic ring, the last share, even though containing the secret value, is indistinguishable from a random value.

Without loss of generality, consider an addition between two parties p_1 and p_2, wanting to securely add their secret inputs v^1 and v^2, respectively. The sampled randomness during secret sharing is denoted as $rand^1$ and $rand^2$. The parties withheld one share and exchanged the other, say s_2^i. Both parties add their locally held shares, that is for $p_1: S^1 = s_1^1 + s_2^2 \mod r = rand^1 + (v^2 - rand^2) \mod r$ and for $p_2: S^2 = s_1^2 + s_2^1 \mod r = rand^2 + (v^1 - rand^1) \mod r$. If they both now recombine these new two shares $R = S^1 + S^2 \mod r = rand^1 + (v^2 - rand^2) + rand^2 + (v^1 - rand^1) \mod r = v^2 + v^1 \mod r$, the randomness cancels out and the clear text sum is revealed. Of course, the two-party case is purely instructional, as knowledge of the result and the own secret value always allows to calculate the secret value of the other party.

The process was tested on three DSF instances representing three different organizations belonging to the same consortium, each containing a small data set of synthetic patient data. The open source code can be found on GitHub[6].

5. Lessons learned (Discussion)

All five previously defined requirements were met by the purposed MPC feasibility query solution. As a research advancement based on the HiGHmed DSF feasibility process, existing advantages such as fully decentralized computation without central components were retained while simultaneously advancing the state-of-the-art by significantly raising the patients' data privacy level and addressing the additional requirements of new use cases, mainly the elimination of the TTP.

The usage of open standards simplifies the integration of local systems, including the translation of cohort queries into a suitable format for each repository. This was an important consideration, as HiGHmed organizations employ a local OpenEHR repository, while NUM institutions may incorporate i2b2[7] data warehouses besides FHIR stores. Using FHIR resources as a linking data model, we provide semantic interoperability and built-in audit capabilities.

Allowing researchers to optionally perform consent checks enables additional use cases, like consent-less epidemiological studies, and creates concise interfaces for the adoption of changing legal consent requirements. In comparison to the TTP-based feasibility query process, this work does currently not support the incorporation of Record Linkage (RL). Solutions for MPC-based TTP-less RL were developed in the HiGHmed consortium [20]. The complexity and performance requirements pose a future challenge when direct integration of RL within the DSF is required. Furthermore, the development of bidirectional communication interfaces is an interesting research possibility for future work.

As no central components are employed and authorization between organizational DSF instances are handled on a pipeline- and framework level, only local user and process authorization is required to perform user authentication. This enables organizations to deploy and integrate authorization and authentication solutions of their own choosing. The complexity of inter-domain user management is avoided.

As MPC only provides input privacy, the output might pose a privacy risk. One example was already described in the "Concept" section, extracting an organization's individual cohort size by performing multiple queries, excluding one organization at a time. We mitigated this specific attack vector by forbidding the selection of individual target organizations. Other attack scenarios might be mitigated using, e.g., rate-limiting. In all cases, an audit trail is maintained by the DSF, thus adversarial behavior is identifiable.

Testing was performed on a setup with three DSF instances representing three organizations operating on small, synthetically generated data sets. While this assures correct operation, optimizing parameter values e.g., timeout durations and retry counts, must be dealt with in real, operating systems. The choice of these parameters are heavily influenced by network- and bandwidth settings, as well as the deployed hardware and firewall specifications.

---

[6] https://github.com/highmed/highmed-processes
[7] https://www.i2b2.org

This work is intended as a pragmatic starting point to introduce MPC protocols and analysis processes into real-world applications. It solves a real-world demand not achievable with traditional distributed computation techniques, while maintaining a reasonable scope.

6. Conclusion

To provide a decentralized feasibility process for calculating multi-centric cohort sizes with highest data privacy guarantees and without a Trusted Third Party, this work proposes a secure Multi-Party Computation based implementation using the open standards BPMN 2.0 and HL7 FHIR R4. The solution is provided as a plugin process to the HiGHmed Data Sharing Framework, allowing the easy usage for all organizations employing the HiGHmed and MII infrastructure. The process is based on the principle of data minimization by avoiding central components and, additionally, allows (optional) consent validation procedures. Identifying data never leaves organizational boundaries and data privacy regulations are acknowledged, even for small (local) cohort sizes, i.e., in rare disease research. By providing a freely available implementation under a permissive open source license, this process can be used outside the HiGHmed consortium and is easily adaptable to specific use cases.

Declarations

Conflict of Interest: The authors declare that there is no conflict of interest.

Contributions of the authors: RW and TK designed, implemented, and tested the processes. HH and CF managed the HiGHmed DSF integration and maintenance. MD and KH led and supervised the project. All authors contributed to the manuscript and substantively revised it. All authors read and approved the final manuscript.

Acknowledgements: This project is funded by the German Federal Ministry of Education and Research (BMBF, grant ids: 01ZZ1802A, 01ZZ1802E, and 01ZZ1802G). It was co-funded by the Deutsche Forschungsgemeinschaft (DFG) – SFB 1119 CROSSING/236615297. Many thanks to Fabian Prasser, Ulrich Sax, and Jürgen Eils for our fruitful discussions. The authors would like to thank all committers that contributed to the open source reference implementation and to test the current release.

References

[1]   M. Grossglauser and H. Saner, "Data-driven healthcare: from patterns to actions," *Eur J Prev Cardiolog*, vol. 21, no. 2_suppl, pp. 14–17, Nov. 2014, doi: 10.1177/2047487314552755.
[2]   A. Shaban-Nejad, M. Michalowski, and D. L. Buckeridge, "Health intelligence: how artificial intelligence transforms population and personalized health," *npj Digital Med*, vol. 1, no. 1, Art. no. 1, Oct. 2018, doi: 10.1038/s41746-018-0058-9.
[3]   H. Hsin *et al.*, "Transforming Psychiatry into Data-Driven Medicine with Digital Measurement Tools," *npj Digital Med*, vol. 1, no. 1, Art. no. 1, Aug. 2018, doi: 10.1038/s41746-018-0046-0.

[4] G. Carra, J. I. F. Salluh, F. J. da Silva Ramos, and G. Meyfroidt, "Data-driven ICU management: Using Big Data and algorithms to improve outcomes," *Journal of Critical Care*, vol. 60, pp. 300–304, Dec. 2020, doi: 10.1016/j.jcrc.2020.09.002.

[5] L. V. Rasmussen, "The Electronic Health Record for Translational Research," *J. of Cardiovasc. Trans. Res.*, vol. 7, no. 6, pp. 607–614, Aug. 2014, doi: 10.1007/s12265-014-9579-z.

[6] P. Knaup, T. M. Deserno, H.-U. Prokosch, and U. Sax, "Implementation of a National Framework to Promote Health Data Sharing," *Yearb Med Inform*, vol. 27, no. 1, pp. 302–304, Aug. 2018, doi: 10.1055/s-0038-1641210.

[7] N. Yüksekogul, N. Meyer, S. Aguduri, A. Merzweiler, and O. Heinze, "ETL-Processes for a medical data integration Center–First experiences from the heidelberg university hospital, 64," *Jahrestagung der Deutschen Gesellschaft für Medizinische Informatik, Biometrie und Epidemiologie (GMDS), DocAbstr*, vol. 112, 2019.

[8] S. Aguduri, A. Merzweiler, N. Yüksekogul, N. Meyer, A. Brandner, and O. Heinze, "Modeling clinical data transformation for a medical data integration center: An openEHR approach, 64," *Jahrestagung der Deutschen Gesellschaft für Medizinische Informatik, Biometrie und Epidemiologie (GMDS), DocAbstr*, vol. 113, 2019.

[9] T. Wendt et al., "Prozessmodelle des Data Sharing im Rahmen der Medizin- informatik-Initiative," AG Data Sharing MI-I, unpublished, 2019.

[10] Taskforce Datenschutz der MII mit Vertretern der Konsortien DIFUTURE, HiGHmed, MIRACUM, SMITH, dem Sprecher der AG Datenschutz der TMF sowie Vertretern der TMF-Geschäftsstelle, "Übergreifendes Datenschutzkonzept der Medizininformatik-Initiative," TF Datenschutz MI-I, unpublished, 2021.

[11] B. Haarbrandt et al., "HiGHmed – An Open Platform Approach to Enhance Care and Research across Institutional Boundaries," *Methods Inf Med*, vol. 57, no. S 01, pp. e66–e81, May 2018, doi: 10.3414/ME18-02-0002.

[12] H. Hund, R. Wettstein, C. M. Heidt, and C. Fegeler, "Executing distributed healthcare and research Processes–The HiGHmed data sharing framework," *Studies in Health Technology and Informatics*, vol. 278, pp. 126–133, 2021.

[13] M. Lablans, E. E. Schmidt, and F.Ückert, "An Architecture for Translational Cancer Research As Exemplified by the German Cancer Consortium," *JCO Clinical Cancer Informatics*, no. 2, pp. 1–8, Dec. 2018, doi: 10.1200/CCI.17.00062.

[14] "Clinical Research Platform: DZHK." https://dzhk.de/en/research/clinical-research/clinical-research-platform/ (accessed Feb. 16, 2022).

[15] R. Wettstein, H. Hund, I. Kobylinski, C. Fegeler, and O. Heinze, "Feasibility queries in distributed Architectures–Concept and implementation in HiGHmed," in *German medical data sciences: Bringing data to life*, IOS Press, 2021, pp. 134–141.

[16] "CODEX | Netzwerk Universitätsmedizin." https://www.netzwerk-universitaetsmedizin.de/projekte/codex (accessed Feb. 16, 2022).

[17] A. C. Yao, "How to generate and exchange secrets," in *27th Annual Symposium on Foundations of Computer Science (sfcs 1986)*, Oct. 1986, pp. 162–167. doi: 10.1109/sfcs.1986.25.

[18] D. Malkhi, N. Nisan, B. Pinkas, and Y. Sella, "Fairplay — A Secure Two-Party Computation System," 2004, p. 17.

[19] O. Goldreich, S. Micali, and A. Wigderson, "How to Play ANY Mental Game," New York, NY, USA, 1987. doi: 10.1145/28395.28420.

[20] S. Stammler et al., "Mainzelliste SecureEpiLinker (MainSEL): Privacy-Preserving Record Linkage using Secure Multi-Party Computation," *Bioinformatics*, 2020, doi: 10.1093/bioinformatics/btaa764.

50

German Medical Data Sciences 2022 - Future Medicine
R. Röhrig et al. (Eds.)
© 2022 The authors and IOS Press.
This article is published online with Open Access by IOS Press and distributed under the terms
of the Creative Commons Attribution Non-Commercial License 4.0 (CC BY-NC 4.0).
doi:10.3233/SHTI220803

Guideline-Based Context-Sensitive Decision Modeling for Melanoma Patients

Catharina Lena BECKMANN[a,1], Georg LODDE[b], Elisabeth LIVINGSTONE[b], Dirk
SCHADENDORF[b], and Britta BÖCKMANN[a,c]

[a] *Department of Computer Science, University of Applied Sciences and Arts Dortmund
(FH Dortmund), 44227 Dortmund, Germany*
[b] *Department of Dermatology, Venereology and Allergology, University Hospital
Essen, 45147 Essen, Germany*
[c] *Institute of Medical Informatics, Biometry and Epidemiology (IMIBE), University
Hospital Essen, 45122 Essen, Germany*

Abstract. Introduction: The provision of knowledge through clinical practice
guidelines and hospital-specific standard operating procedures (SOPs) is ubiquitous
in the medical context and in the treatment of melanoma patients. However, these
knowledge sources are only available in unstructured text form and without any
contextual link to real patient data. The aim of our project is to give a modeled
decision support for the next treatment step based on the actual data and position of
a patient. **Methods:** First, we identified passages for qualified decision-making
necessary at the point of care from the SOP for melanoma. Thereby, the patient-
specific contextual reference data at decision points was considered in parallel and
represented by FHIR (Fast Healthcare Interoperability Resource) resources. The
decision algorithm was then formalized using BPMN modeling with FHIR
annotations. Validation was provided by medical experts, dermatooncologists from
University Hospital Essen. **Results:** The resulting BPMN model is presented here
with the diagnostic procedure of sentinel lymph node excision as the example
snippet from the whole algorithm. Each decision point is edited with FHIR resources
covering the patient data and preparing the context sensitivity of the model.
Conclusion: Modeling guideline-based information into a decision algorithm that
can be presented at the point of care with contextual reference, may have the
potential to support patient-specific clinical decision-making. For patients from a
certain status like in the metastatic setting modeling becomes highly tailored to
specific patient cases, alternative and individualized treatment options.

Keywords. Clinical Practice Guideline, Clinical Pathway, Clinical Decision-
Making, BPMN, Patient-Specific Modeling, Malignant Melanoma

1. Introduction

Clinical practice guidelines (e.g., the national S3 guideline on the diagnosis, treatment,
and follow-up of melanoma [1]) and hospital-specific SOPs (e.g., the hospital-specific
document *SOP Malignes Melanom*[2] [Malignant Melanoma] of the Department of
Dermatology of the University Hospital Essen) generally provide useful knowledge for

---

[1] Corresponding Author. Catharina Lena Beckmann, E-mail: catharina.beckmann@fh-dortmund.de.

[2] Livingstone E, Zimmer L, Schadendorf D. SOP Malignes Melanom. 2020 Apr. ID: 11365. Unpublished,
internal hospital document.

evidence-based care and are used alongside clinical pathways to bring this knowledge into clinical practice. By incorporating all elements of systematic reviews and meta-analyses, S3 guidelines provide the guidelines with the highest evidence base and the highest methodological quality in the medical field [2]. Many guidelines provide treatment recommendations over the entire course of a disease, and SOPs contain the AWMF S3 guideline shortened to the essential treatment steps and provide step-by-step instructions [3] for hospital-specific treatment processes. For this work, we used the document *SOP Malignes Melanom*[2], a shortened version of the *national S3 guideline on the diagnosis, treatment, and follow-up of melanoma* adapted to hospital-specific processes and longer in content than usual SOPs.

To bring evidence-based knowledge into clinical practice, related works map guidelines into FHIR: The EBMonFHIR project extends FHIR to evidence-based medical data and aims to create interoperability for clinical research and clinical care recommendations [4] and the FHIR Clinical Guidelines Implementation Guide (CPG-IG) codifies clinical guidelines to provide evidence-based and best practice recommendations at the point of care [5]. While both works demonstrate how guideline information can be mapped into FHIR and brought to the point of care, they currently do not consider the contextual link between guidelines and SOPs as knowledge sources and the specific patient and physician user. Proper utilization of this knowledge is elaborate and costly as identifying appropriate guideline- or SOP-based information linked to a specific patient context requires a time-consuming search by physicians [6]. Reasons for this are the unstructured information base and missing links of existing modeling and mapping procedures for guidelines to a specific patient or user context from the clinical perspective.

Therefore, this work aims to enhance modeling in a way that the clinical context as well as the available data of a specific patient are considered and used automatically in a later step to give context-sensitive decision support. Specifically, we establish the contextual link between information from the SOP document and actual patient data so that the history and medical status can be identified automatically. This data is provided by the "Smart Hospital Information Platform" (SHIP)[3] of the University Medicine Essen, which was set up for research purposes and contains all clinical information transferred into FHIR format. For the SHIP data, the following clinical information systems serve as sources: Hospital Information System (HIS), Radiological Information System (RIS), three Picture Archiving and Communication Systems (PACS), Patient-Recorded Outcomes (PRO), Laboratory Information System (LIS) and Pathology Information System (ISP).

We selected malignant melanoma, the most dangerous and aggressive skin tumor due to its propensity for metastatic spread [8], as the medical model. The presentation of the modeling here focusses on a snippet of the whole algorithm – the pathway for the sentinel lymph node excision (SLNE) diagnostic procedure as sentinel lymph node status is one of the most important prognostic factors in early-stage melanoma [8][9]. SLNE is initially recommended for all patients with any of the following: tumor thickness between 0.75 mm and 1 mm and present risk factors as ulceration, mitotic rate >=1 mitosis and patient age < 40 years, tumor thickness greater than 1 mm and no ulceration present, tumor thickness greater than 1 mm to 4 mm and ulceration present, or tumor thickness greater than 4 mm and ulceration present. Therefore, the indication for or against a SLNE is relevant for a large proportion of melanoma patients.

---

[3] SHIP: see [7, p. 294]

The whole clinical algorithm contains 53 different decision points, 7 of which are presented in the SLNE section.

2. Methods

To visualize and harmonize the knowledge from the hospital-specific document *SOP Malignes Melanom* as a graphical workflow, we first manually identified the passages necessary for qualified decision-making in the document. For correct identification of medical knowledge, but also for the purpose of iterative inclusion of physician-specific context, the identification step was accompanied and validated by a dermatooncologist of the University Hospital Essen. To ensure that the identified information reflected the level of experience of physicians of all experience levels, but initially of junior physician, the information identification process was initially performed in a very small-step manner in collaboration with a junior physician and checked for medical correctness. The information modules classified as relevant were marked as such directly in the corresponding knowledge source.

For the marked information modules we then additionally identified necessary FHIR (Fast Healthcare Interoperability Resources)[4] resources representing patient data needed for decisions. Thereby the contextual link between the SOP document containing guideline-based knowledge and real patient data was established.

Final modeling was performed with Business Process Model And Notation (BPMN)[5] modeling elements using the open-source modeling tool Camunda Modeler[6]. The modeling was validated by two dermatooncologists of different qualifications (one senior physician, one junior physician); initially iteratively by the junior physician and after the first modeling draft was created by the senior physician. The context reference at decision points was realized via data storage elements. The element names refer to FHIR resources within SHIP.

Figure 1 illustrates the described procedure summarized in graphical form.

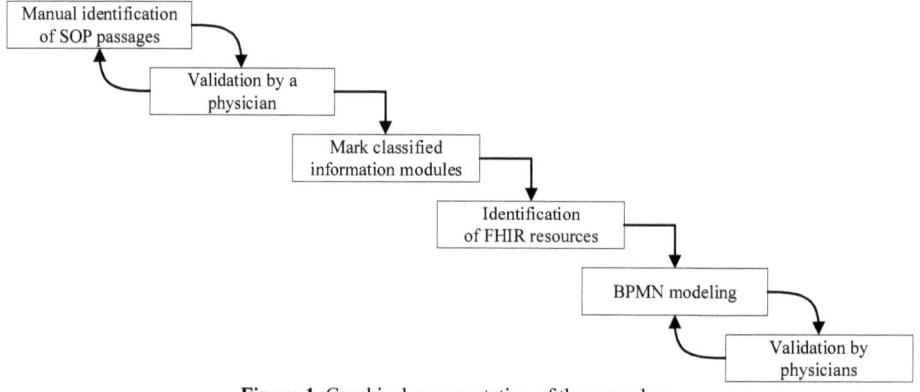

Figure 1. Graphical representation of the procedure

---

[4] FHIR standard: https://www.hl7.org/fhir/ (18.02.2022)

[5] BPMN platform: https://www.omg.org/spec/BPMN/2.0/ (18.02.2022)

[6] Camunda Modeler platform: https://camunda.com/de/platform/modeler/ (20.04.2022)

3. Results

Compared with the overall modeling of the entire melanoma treatment, the SLNE section presented as an example in this article represents only a small part of the overall modeling. To quantify the dimension of the overall modeling versus the SLNE excerpt, we compared the number of selected modeling elements utilized in the excerpt to the entire modeling below: The greatest consistency in modeling elements was found in tasks (n=17 of 125; 14%), followed by subprocesses (n=2 of 17; 12%), exclusive gateways (n=13 of 105; 12%), and parallel gateways (n=2 of 40; 5%). This exemplary comparison of selected modeling elements gives an idea of the scope and power of the entire modeled information base *SOP Malignes Melanom*.

The resulting manual extraction of the information modules from the hospital-specific document *SOP Malignes Melanom* is exemplified in Figure 2 using the indication of the diagnostic procedure SLNE.

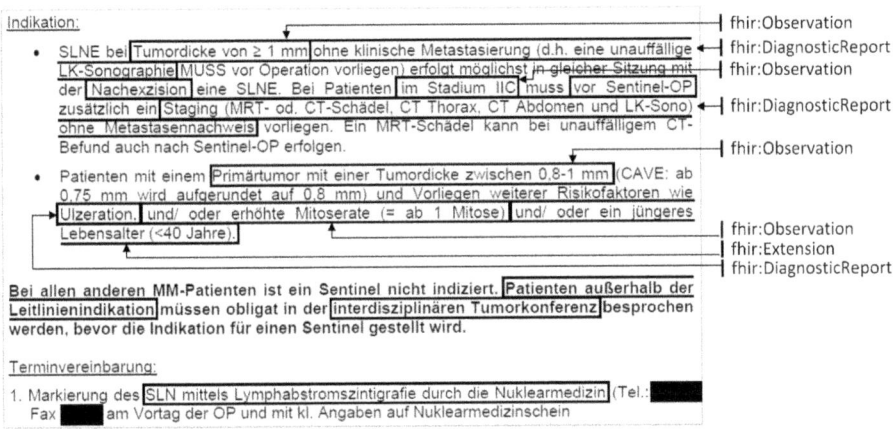

Figure 2. Annotated screenshot of a section of the chapter "Sentinel-Lymphnode-Exzision (SLNE)" from the document *SOP Malignes Melanom*[2] *[Malignant Melanoma]* (see [2], p. 14).

The manual extraction provides the classified content of the information base according to their data relevance. The relevant passages were framed and the corresponding FHIR resource was noted simultaneously in the information base. For example, the patient's tumor thickness [Tumordicke] is stored in the FHIR resource Observation.

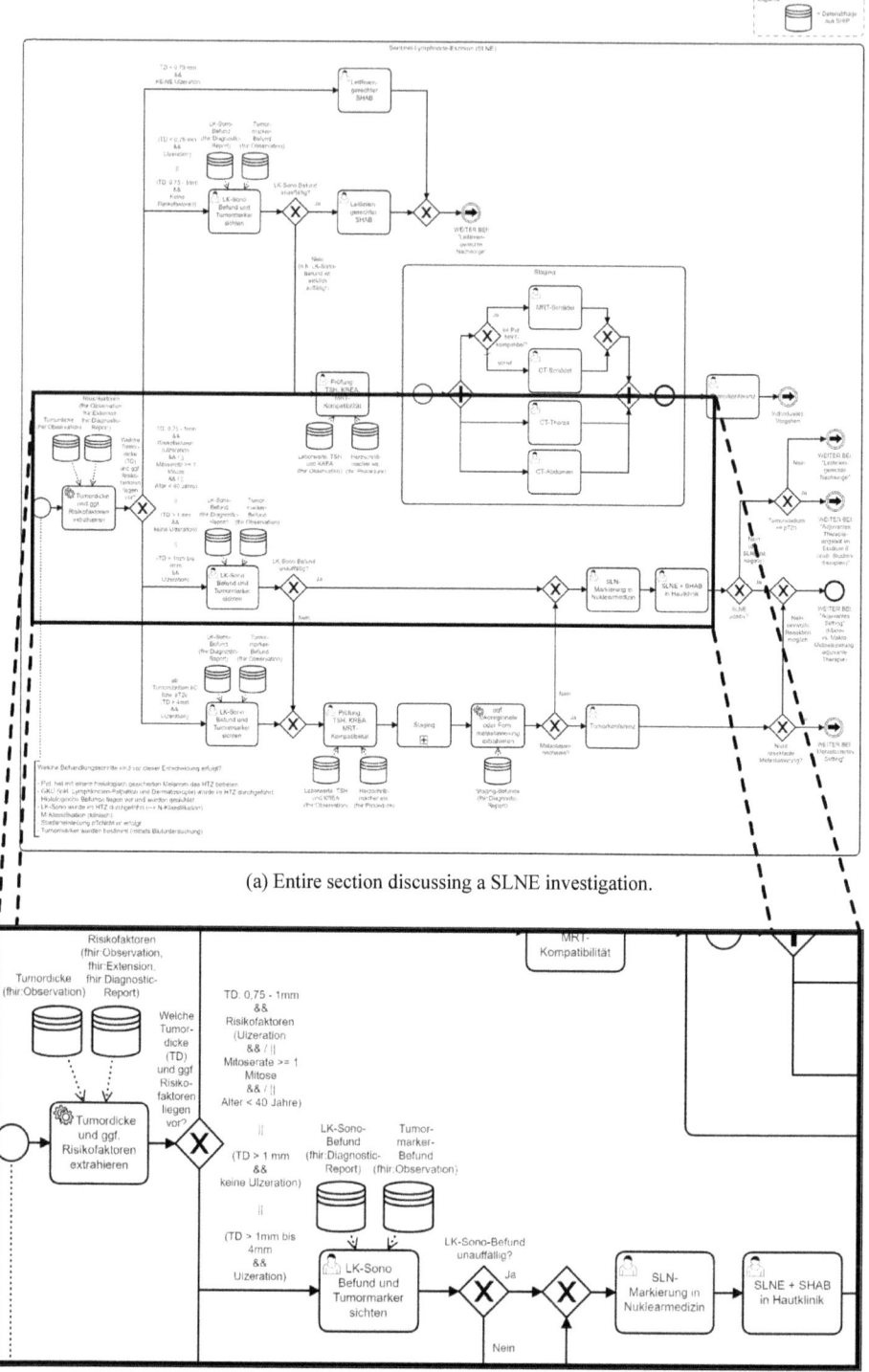

(a) Entire section discussing a SLNE investigation.

(b) Main Pathway in which the SLNE is carried out (see User Task "SLNE + SHAB in Hautklinik").

Figure 3. BPMN representation of the SLNE section.

Figure 3 shows the SLNE subprocess as BPMN modeling. To understand the temporal treatment flow of the modeling, we added the process steps that temporally precede this modeling excerpt (the SLNE) as an annotation to the start state. Depending on the tumor thickness of the patient's primary tumor and the risk factors, SLNE is then performed or not. For a patient with a tumor thickness greater 1.0 mm, no ulceration and inconspicuous lymph node sonography findings (see first two identified information modules in Figure 2), the BPMN modeling indicates that SLNE will be performed (see User Task "SLNE + SHAB in Hautklinik" in Figure 3). The contextual reference prepared in Figure 2 by sideways annotations, i.e., the links between the knowledge of the information base and the real patient data, was represented in the modeling by data storage elements with the label *[data needed for the next decision-making] (fhir:[FHIR Resource])*. These FHIR resources are employed to generate context-sensitive decision recommendations based on the query data when the modelled algorithm is passed later.

Extraction and modeling of all information modules, including parallel contextual reference to real patient data using FHIR resources, was performed for the complete information base *SOP Malignes Melanom* in the same manner as shown for SLNE.

4. Discussion

In this work, we presented BPMN modeling for evidence-based medicine with integrated contextual reference to real patient data annotated in FHIR. The modeling excerpt presented will be useful for the treatment of roughly 155 patient cases per year of the Department of Dermatology of the University Hospital Essen. These patient cases are divided into approximately 125 patient cases per year with an indication for SLNE, for which this modeling can be utilized, and approximately 30 patient cases who only require a wide margin excision, and for whom the modeling indicates that they do not require a SLNE.

The transfer of the classified information modules to BPMN modeling shows, using the SLNE as an example, that modeling as a decision algorithm has limited value beyond a specific degree of detail. Above this level, modeling becomes in this case highly tailored to specific patient cases and alternative treatment options due to more and more individualized and specific oncological treatment options. In the modeling extract, this is exemplified to patients with tumor thickness less than 0.75 mm and ulceration present, or patients with tumor thickness between 0.75 and 1 mm without risk factors, each with conspicuous lymph node sonography findings (see event "individuelles Vorgehen" [individual approach] in Figure 3). For patients in the metastatic setting, this limited value occurs significantly more frequently. Therefore, we focused on the main treatment performed as defined in the hospital-specific SOP document rather than each optional treatment alternative. To double-check which optional treatment suggestions described in the SOP document, we consulted the S3 guideline.

The contextual reference between the information base and real patient data was established using FHIR resources to provide FHIR-oriented data access at the decision points in the further project. Compared to related projects mapping guidelines to FHIR, this contextual link to real patient has not yet been established (see [4][5]). For data that is so far not described in standard FHIR resources, extensions will be used. In addition, for FHIR-oriented data access, quality, readiness, and completeness of SHIP data is essential to use it in its entirety. This verification is currently being carried out in a parallel work.

Although the modeling presented may offer advantages such as the accurate representation of information at the point of care, its form needs to be evaluated subsequently. It remains to be investigated whether pure modeling of treatment steps supports physicians in decision-making during melanoma treatment or whether additional – possibly textual – information is needed. The additional information would then also be incorporated into the modeling.

5. Conclusion

By providing physicians with the information needed for the subsequent treatment steps in a clear, standardized, and guideline-compliant way, as well as considering the contextual reference to the individual patient, we intend to make a significant contribution to rapid and patient-specific medical decision-making for melanoma patients in the clinical setting, for which this work represents the first step through its context-sensitive decision modeling.

The modeling presented illustrates a modeling approach to potentially better present contextual guideline information for the treatment of malignant melanoma at the point of care, specifically for the indication for or against a SLNE, and to better embed guideline information into the patient workflow. Using the Guide2Treat[7] software, the information could thus be queried context-sensitively from the modeling in later project phases.

The modeling created based on an unstructured information source, which was presented as an example using the SLNE subprocess, shows the current state of modeling initially represents only the preliminary work for a clinical decision support system (CDSS). In a further step, we will integrate this model into everyday clinical practice. Thereby, we are aware that precautions, such as criteria for qualification as a medical device or as medical device software, must be taken in the general application of CDSS in clinical routine; however, we will work retrospectively as part of this research. We will investigate whether the modeling developed in theory needs to be modified for its use in everyday practice and at which points in the modeling there are deviations between theory and clinical practice. The next steps are to simulate the approximately 2,000 data sets from SHIP and verify the modeling against those data sets.

---

[7] Guide2Treat software: https://ieee-dataport.org/documents/guide2treat-software (23.02.2022)

Declarations

Ethical vote: Ethik-Kommission der Medizinischen Fakultät der Universität Duisburg-Essen, Prof. Dr. U. Schara-Schmidt, 21-10391-BO, 02.12.2021

Conflict of Interest: The authors declare, that there is no conflict of interest.

Author contributions:
CB, BB: conception of the work, data aquisition and interpretation;
CB, GL: study design, data analysis and interpretation;
GL, EL, DS: monitoring and validation of the information identification process and the BPMN modeling;
CB: writing the manuscript;
BB, EL: substantial revising of the manuscript.
All authors approved the manuscript in the submitted version and take responsibility for the scientific integrity of the work.

Acknowledgement: This work was funded by a PhD grant from the DFG Research Training Group 2535 Knowledge- and data-based personalization of medicine at the point of care (WisPerMed), University of Duisburg-Essen, Germany.

References

[1] Leitlinienprogramm Onkologie (Deutsche Krebsgesellschaft, Deutsche Krebshilfe, AWMF). Diagnostik, Therapie und Nachsorge des Melanoms. Langversion 3.3. 2020 Jul. AWMF Registernummer: 032/024OL. http://www.leitlinienprogramm-onkologie.de/leitlinien/melanom/ http://www.leitlinienprogramm-onkologie.de/leitlinien/melanom/ (accessed February 15, 2022).
[2] AWMF Leitlinien. Available at: https://www.awmf.org/leitlinien.html (accessed 25 February 2022).
[3] Lödel S, Ostgathe C, Heckel M, et al. Standard Operating Procedures (SOPs) for Palliative Care in German Comprehensive Cancer Centers - an evaluation of the implementation status. BMC palliative care. 2020 May; 19(1): 62. doi: 10.1186/s12904-020-00565-6.
[4] EBMonFHIR. HL7 Confluence Page. https://confluence.hl7.org/display/CDS/EBMonFHIR (accessed May 04, 2022).
[5] FHIR Clinical Guidelines. http://hl7.org/fhir/uv/cpg/ (accessed May 04, 2022).
[6] Becker M, Kasper S, Böckmann B, Jöckel KH, Virchow I. Natural language processing of German clinical colorectal cancer notes for guideline-based treatment evaluation. Int J Med Inform. 2019 Jul; 127:141-146. doi: 10.1016/j.ijmedinf.2019.04.022.
[7] Tewes R. Mutige Zukunft der Personalentwicklung im Gesundheitswesen. Innovative Personalentwicklung im In- und Ausland. Springer, Berlin, Heidelberg. 2021 Nov; 285-335. doi: 10.1007/978-3-662-62977-2.
[8] Gershenwald JE, Scolyer RA, Hess KR, Sondak VK, Long GV, Ross MI, Lazar AJ, Faries MB, Kirkwood JM, McArthur GA, Haydu LE, Eggermont AMM, Flaherty KT, Balch CM, Thompson JF; for members of the American Joint Committee on Cancer Melanoma Expert Panel and the International Melanoma Database and Discovery Platform. Melanoma staging: Evidence-based changes in the American Joint Committee on Cancer eighth edition cancer staging manual. CA Cancer J Clin. 2017 Nov; 67(6):472-492. doi: 10.3322/caac.21409.
[9] Mays MP, Martin RC, Burton A, Ginter B, Edwards MJ, Reintgen DS, Ross MI, Urist MM, Stromberg AJ, McMasters KM, Scoggins CR. Should all patients with melanoma between 1 and 2 mm Breslow thickness undergo sentinel lymph node biopsy? Cancer. 2010 Mar 15; 116(6):1535-44. doi: 10.1002/cncr.24895.

German Medical Data Sciences 2022 - Future Medicine
R. Röhrig et al. (Eds.)
© 2022 The authors and IOS Press.

doi:10.3233/SHTI220804

CODEX Meets RACOON - A Concept for Collaborative Documentation of Clinical and Radiological COVID-19 Data

Marvin SCHMIDT[a,1], Sebastian GEBAUER[a], Annette BARTHOLMES[b], Dennis
KADIOGLU[a,b], Jens KLEESIEK[c], Bernd HAMM[d], Thomas J. VOGL[e], Tobias
PENZKOFER[d], Andreas Michael BUCHER[e] and Holger STORF[a,b]

[a] *Institute of Medical Informatics, Goethe University Frankfurt, University Hospital Frankfurt, Frankfurt am Main, Germany*
[b] *Data Integration Center, University Hospital Frankfurt, Frankfurt am Main, Germany*
[c] *Institute for AI in Medicine (IKIM), University Hospital Essen, Essen, Germany*
[d] *Department of Radiology, Charité Universitätsmedizin Berlin, Berlin, Germany*
[e] *Department of Diagnostic and Interventional Radiology, University Hospital Frankfurt, Frankfurt am Main, Germany*

Abstract. Within the scope of the two NUM projects CODEX and RACOON we developed a preliminary technical concept for documenting clinical and radiological COVID-19 data in a collaborative approach and its preceding findings of a requirement analysis. At first, we provide an overview of NUM and its two projects CODEX and RACOON including the GECCO data set. Furthermore, we demonstrate the foundation for the increased collaboration of both projects, which was additionally supported by a survey conducted at University Hospital Frankfurt. Based on the survey results mint Lesion™, developed by Mint Medical and used at all project sites within RACOON, was selected as the "Electronic Data Capture" (EDC) system for CODEX. Moreover, to avoid duplicate entry of GECCO data into both EDC systems, an early effort was made to consider a collaborative and efficient technical approach to reduce the workload for the medical documentalists. As a first effort we present a preliminary technical concept representing the current and possible future data workflow of CODEX and RACOON. This concept includes a software component to synchronize GECCO data sets between the two EDC systems using the HL7 FHIR standard. Our first approach of a collaborative use of an EDC system and its medical documentalists could be beneficial in combination with the presented synchronization component for all participating project sites of CODEX and RACOON with regard to an overall reduced documentation workload.

Keywords. COVID-19, CODEX, RACOON, EDC, clinical documentation

1. Introduction

As part of an initiative of the "German Federal Ministry of Education and Research" (BMBF), the German COVID-19 Research "Network of University Medicine" (NUM) was founded. The goal of this network of all German university hospitals is to improve

---

[1] Corresponding Author, Marvin Schmidt, Institute of Medical Informatics, Goethe University Frankfurt, University Hospital Frankfurt, Theodor-Stern-Kai 7, 60590 Frankfurt am Main, Germany; E-mail: marvin.schmidt@kgu.de.

the general availability of relevant routine and research data as needed for thirteen innovative research projects which should contribute to the management of the pandemic and thus enable the best possible treatment of COVID-19 patients. Accordingly, the network also takes into account the necessary digitalization and finally promotes "Pandemic Preparedness" [1]. In addition to the network, the "German Corona Consensus Data Set" (GECCO) provides another foundation for collaboration in the wake of the COVID-19 pandemic. The GECCO data set describes 83 data items grouped by different categories such as anamnesis/risk factors, imaging and demographics. This consensus data set provides scientists with a research foundation, related to key clinical parameters of COVID-19 [2].

1.1. CODEX and RACOON

The "COVID-19 Data Exchange Platform" (CODEX) is one of the thirteen NUM projects. It is mainly focused on the development of a secure nationwide, interoperable and privacy-compliant research infrastructure for the storage and provision of COVID-19 research datasets [3]. The architecture of CODEX is structured into decentralized nodes (NUM nodes), which are mainly operated by the "Data Integration Centers" (DIZ). These decentralized parts of the platform use existing infrastructures of the "Medical Informatics Initiative" (MII). In addition, there is also a central component (CODEX platform) which supports data provision and use. The platform processes the collected data in the format of the nationwide coordinated GECCO data set [4]. An integral requirement for the storage of the data in the CODEX platform, besides the local pseudonymization, is the provision of the MII Broad Consent, which is ultimately the corresponding consent of the patients for the further processing of their data. The Broad Consent is also the current, coordinated legal basis for the decentralized collection, aggregation and centralized release of health data for research in NUM [5]. If both of these conditions are met, the data is passed on with the cooperation of several components and organizations such as the "GECCO Transfer HUB" (GTH) and the "federated Trusted Third Party" (fTTP). The GTH is responsible for transmitting the medical data (MDAT) distributed by the DIZ to the CODEX Platform. It exchanges the local DIZ pseudonym (DIZ PSN) for the central CODEX pseudonym (CODEX PSN) provided by the fTTP. This ensures a consistent separation of medical data and patient-identifying data (IDAT) [5].

A nationwide infrastructure is also being established within the "Radiological Cooperative Network" (RACOON) for the structured collection of radiological data from COVID-19 cases [6]. For this purpose, all 36 university radiology departments from Germany have joined forces to face the challenges of the COVID-19 pandemic from a radiological perspective [7]. The infrastructure in the RACOON project is based in particular on a nationwide server system with network nodes (RACOON-NODE) at all German university hospitals. The preliminary work, project structure and design were in large parts contributed by the project partner now affiliated with IKIM. The sites in Frankfurt and Berlin are in the lead for project organization and coordination across all partner sites. The RACOON infrastructure represents an integration of the decentralized and centralized (RACOON-CENTRAL) components into a powerful overall concept. RACOON enables a consolidation of the collected diagnostic data within a standardized data model based on the GECCO data set for collaborative research projects. Within RACOON-CENTRAL, both anonymized data sets as well as structured reports of findings can be generated. The data protection description for RACOON specifies that personal data are only processed locally within the respective clinic network under the sole control of the responsible authority by an approved medical device. Outside the clinic network (especially on RACOON Central), only anonymized data is transmitted and processed [8].

1.2. Collaboration between CODEX and RACOON at UKF

The University Hospital Frankfurt (UKF) is involved in seven of the 13 NUM research projects, three of which are coordinated by Frankfurt in the overall network. Since the start of NUM it has always been a primary goal to foster synergies and increase cooperation between the projects at the UKF [9]. Since both in CODEX and RACOON "Electronic Data Capture" (EDC) systems are used for follow-up documentation of clinical parameters, the question arose early on how to approach this matter as efficiently and collaboratively as possible for both projects. The primary goal of this paper was to provide a first preliminary technical concept for documenting clinical and radiological COVID-19 data for the two NUM projects in a collaborative and efficient approach, to ultimately minimize redundant documentation and therefore provide an additional technical and organizational effort for them. We present the main outcomes of the preceding requirement analysis, the resulting preliminary concept and its findings which could be relevant for other participating sites.

2. Methods

2.1. Software used within CODEX and RACOON

"Extract, Transform, Load" (ETL) processes are used within CODEX to transform the collected data into a standardized format. In addition, medical documentalists use an EDC system for follow-up documentation of missing parameters [10]. For CODEX, the EDC systems "Research Electronic Data Capture" (REDCap) and "Data Integration System" (DIS) were provided by the national project management with the further option to use other systems [11,12]. The documented data in the EDC system are in "Clinical Data Interchange Standards Consortium -Operational Data Model CDISC ODM" format. This format is primarily used for EDC systems. It consists of a structured XML file that supports the platform-independent exchange and archiving of research data [13]. The CDISC ODM data are then transformed using the ODM2FHIR application, which is part of a software node (NUM Node v2) that was implemented by the various CODEX project partners and made available to all sites [14]. During this process, they are transformed into HL7 "Fast Healthcare Interoperability Resources" (FHIR) resources. This standard offers high interoperability as an exchange format [15]. In this node, important adjustments such as transformation into standardized formats and the general pseudonymization of the data are performed [16]. After complete transformation, the research data and their corresponding pseudonyms are then transmitted to the central CODEX platform via the GTH and the fTTP in a privacy-compliant and pseudonymized manner and thus made available to the researchers [10]. Within RACOON, the "mint Lesion™" software from industrial partner "Mint Medical GmbH" (Heidelberg) is used at each project site. mint Lesion™ is a certified medical software for the assessment of radiological images. The software is primarily aimed at radiologists, physicians and researchers for context-supported reporting of findings using the integrated EDC component and for structured reporting in radiology [7].

2.2. Requirements analysis

In order to promote synergies between the different NUM projects, a requirements analysis with the involved partners at the Frankfurt site was conducted at the beginning of the projects. For this purpose, the scope of the required clinical parameters was relevant, in order to identify the greatest possible overlap between the local NUM projects, to then start a more in-depth collaboration. Accordingly, a survey was conducted in late 2020 together with the DIZ, which aimed to capture the relevant data elements of the GECCO data and the considered cohorts of the corresponding NUM projects at the Frankfurt site. The survey was conducted as a multi-page questionnaire which was send to the participating NUM projects. Additionally, for CODEX a decision had to be made in favor of an EDC system, which would be used to complete the documentation and follow-up documentation of the GECCO data in the further course of the project. During initial discussions regarding the decision about the EDC system it became clear, that in addition to REDCap and DIS the EDC component of mint Lesion™ could also be used for CODEX. This consideration emerged during previous discussions regarding the recruitment of medical documentalists, which are essential in both projects to perform follow-up documentation of clinical and radiological parameters. Moreover, to avoid duplicate entry of GECCO data into both EDC systems, an early effort was made to consider a collaborative and efficient technical approach to reduce the workload of medical documentalists.

3. Results

3.1. Requirements analysis

The evaluated results of this multi-page questionnaire revealed at a broad level, that the data required by all projects were nearly consistent. However, on finer inspection, heterogeneity was nevertheless apparent with regard to the data required as well as the definition of the patient cohorts required in each case. The highest overlap of all projects here was observed for RACOON and CODEX. While CODEX covers the entire GECCO data set, only an intersection of the data set is relevant in RACOON. It is worth mentioning, that RACOON is one of the three NUM projects with the project lead in Frankfurt, together with the Berlin site. Based on these findings, increased cooperation between CODEX and RACOON at the Frankfurt site for the further course of the projects appeared to be highly reasonable. Therefore, a "pool" of medical documentalists, consisting of several employees working for CODEX and RACOON was established.

In addition, after reviewing all available EDC systems presented in CODEX, the decision was made in favor of mint Lesion™. Mint Medical has made the necessary additions to mint Lesion™ for its intended use in CODEX. This included support for a CDISC ODM importer for uploading the various patient data, which was adapted to the CODEX data dictionary. A CDISC ODM exporter was integrated for further processing of the data in the software pipeline.

3.2. Preliminary technical concept

As a first preliminary concept, a draft software architecture (see Figure 1.) was developed, that depicts the currently planned data workflow for CODEX (upper part). Integrated here is a future workflow for RACOON (lower part), which includes a future software component for synchronizing GECCO data sets between the two EDC systems using the HL7 FHIR standard and a HAPI FHIR server.

Within CODEX, the clinical parameters are first extracted from a mirror system of the Frankfurt hospital information system (KIS) ORBIS, an Oracle database, using special SQL queries. Subsequently, these unprocessed raw data are converted from a CSV file into the required CDISC ODM format using a self-implemented ETL process (SQL2ODM). Once the data is in this format, it can be loaded into the mint Lesion™ platform. Within the EDC component of mint Lesion™, medical documentalists can then perform a follow-up documentation of missing GECCO dataset parameters. The fully documented dataset can then be exported via the mint Lesion™ exporter in the CDISC ODM format. Afterwards this exported dataset is transformed into HL7 FHIR format through another ETL process (ODM2FHIR) [14]. Within NUM Node v2, a number of modifications are performed including complete pseudonymization of the data. After the ETL process, the data is available in the HL7 FHIR format which can then be loaded into a deployed HAPI FHIR server. Subsequently, the pseudonymized data is transferred to the CODEX platform via the GTH in a privacy-compliant manner and thus made available to the user. In addition, the GTH exchanges the local DIZ PSN for the central CODEX PSN provided by the fTTP. This ensures consistent separation of MDAT and IDAT [5].

If a patient is registered in both systems, parameters and data already collected in CODEX mint Lesion™ can then be synchronized bidirectionally between RACOON and CODEX. The first approach for this is currently the synchronization of FHIR resources within the HAPI FHIR server. Here, a corresponding FHIR component would have to be integrated into mint Lesion™. After a synchronization of the GECCO data set from CODEX, an exchange of the RACOON relevant data sets can take place. The relevant data can then be loaded into the RACOON mint Lesion™. After the follow-up documentation, the anonymized data can be further processed to be ultimately loaded into RACOON-CENTRAL.

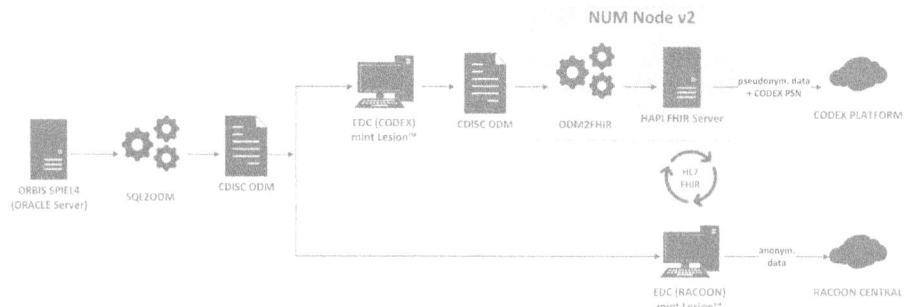

Figure 1. Preliminary technical concept

4. Discussion

One of the main arguments for choosing mint Lesion™ as the EDC system for CODEX was, that in comparison to the other available EDC systems REDCap and DIS, mint Lesion™ offers the advantage that the medical documentalists from the established pool only have to be trained in one system and not in multiple ones, which could ultimately save time and resources. In addition, the documentalists can exchange valuable experience with each other when using the system. Accordingly, synergies were used to efficiently utilize the resources of the medical documentalists for both projects. On the other hand, it must be mentioned here that if REDCap or DIS had been chosen, the general readiness and availability in CODEX would have been faster, since these systems are officially supported and selected in advance by the national project management [10]. mint Lesion™ had to be extended (CDISC ODM importer/exporter) for full use in CODEX in order to meet all project requirements. Another organizational challenge in the preliminary stages of the project was finding suitable and qualified medical documentalists.

Among the technical challenges of the presented concept is, of course, the technical feasibility. Since these projects are nationwide, a large number of stakeholders and locations have to be considered [1]. After a potential implementation, this technical concept could be a useful extension between the two projects in the future. Above all, it should be noted that it has both organizational and technical benefits. The transfer of unprocessed raw data from the KIS is therefore also handled in the same manner for both systems. This could prevent redundant data documentation, which could ultimately reduce the workload and also prevent potential errors while documenting. It is intended that the presented concept prospectively will be implemented by industrial partner Mint Medical. Initial consultations on such a synchronization have already been held with technical managers at Mint Medical. It would thus be an extension of the close collaboration that already existed prior to this paper. The mentioned first possible solution using the HL7 FHIR standard and the HAPI FHIR Server is only one of the suggestions how it could be solved technically.

Despite all the advantages mentioned, the potential difficulties and barriers of such an implementation should not be disregarded because in this context data privacy is crucial. Since these are two projects with different patient cohorts and data scopes, it is necessary that the adopted data privacy concepts in both projects must also be thoroughly reviewed for possible compliance. Prior to such a consolidation, these would naturally have to be reapproved by the corresponding data protection authority because both projects involve sensitive patient data.

The potential developers of such a synchronization component would therefore have to be in close contact with the project managers of both projects in order to coordinate the entire project adequately, which could be challenging due to the size of both projects. Overall, it became apparent during the initial implementation phase that the above-mentioned organizational and technical barriers ultimately prevented the concept from being implemented. The actual benefit of the technical concept presented can only be fully assessed in the future after its first prototypical implementation. In the further course, a more in-depth discussion on the feasibility of such a collaborative data documentation with regard to the data protection admissibility of both projects is inevitable. However, the benefits of the concept could outweigh the expressed concerns, so it is recommended to continue working actively on its implementation. This concept is also expandable, so that other NUM projects can be integrated into the infrastructure and synergies can be used more intensively.

5. Conclusion

All in all, the results of the requirement analysis including the resulting preliminary technical concept presented here show large potential for improved collaboration between CODEX and RACOON in the future. The further findings, such as the adoption of Mint Medical's mint Lesion™ as the EDC system for CODEX and, the creation of a medical documentalists pool for both projects, show that beneficial collaboration is possible despite divergent project aims. The presented findings could therefore be helpful for other participating project sites. Within the follow-up project of CODEX called "CODEX+" are important efforts for deeper cooperation between all NUM projects, such as "Work Package 3.3 Integration with other NUM projects". In Conclusion, the results of this paper can serve as a first good approach to avoid duplication of effort and data entry to ultimately bring both projects closer together. The presented concept of such a data synchronization between the two projects could have great potential due to the reduced documentation workload for the medical documentalists. Furthermore, this solution could be rolled out to other participating sites of CODEX and RACOON to adequately support both projects.

Acknowledgements

CODEX and RACOON are funded in context of NUM by the German Federal Ministry of Education and Research (BMBF). Funding reference number: 01KX2021 (BMBF)

We thank both teams of CODEX and RACOON as well as Mint Medical GmbH (Heidelberg), especially Johannes Kast, Thomas Massier and Dominik Golz for their past and ongoing effort in regards to the support and further development of mint Lesion™.

Declarations

Conflict of Interest: The authors declare, that there is no conflict of interest.

Contributions of the authors: MS and SG contributed to the development of the presented preliminary technical concept. MS, SG, AB, DK, JK, TP, AMB and HS contributed to the overall workflow and the project organization. All authors contributed to drafting and revising this manuscript.

References

[1]   Netzwerk Universitätsmedizin. Netzwerk Universitätsmedizin, Home | Netzwerk Universitätsmedizin [Internet]. [cited 2022 Feb 21]. Available from: https://www.netzwerk-universitaetsmedizin.de/

[2]   Sass J, Bartschke A, Lehne M, Essenwanger A, Rinaldi E, Rudolph S, et al. The German Corona Consensus Dataset (GECCO): a standardized dataset for COVID-19 research in university medicine

and beyond. BMC Med Inform Decis Mak. 2020 Dec 21;20(1):341. DOI: 10.1186/s12911-020-01374-w.

[3]   Netzwerk Universitätsmedizin. CODEX | Netzwerk Universitätsmedizin [Internet]. [cited 2022 Feb 18]. Available from: https://www.netzwerk-universitaetsmedizin.de/projekte/codex

[4]   Ingenerf J. Netzwerk Universitätsmedizin Umsetzungskonzept für den Aufbau einer COVID-19 Data Exchange Plattform (CODEX) [Internet]. [cited 2022 Feb 25]. Available from: https://www.imi.uni-luebeck.de/forschung/p51-netzwerk-uni-medizin.html

[5]   Bahls T, Hampf C, Bialke M, Hoffmann W, Universitätsmedizin Greifswald. Lösungsbaustein fTTP (federated Trusted Third Party) als ein Enabler für vernetzte medizinische Forschung mit dezentraler Datenhaltung [Internet]. [cited 2022 May 11]. Available from: https://www.ths-greifswald.de/wp-content/uploads/2021/11/2021-09-10-fTTP-fact-sheet.pdf

[6]   Netzwerk Universitätsmedizin. RACOON | Netzwerk Universitätsmedizin [Internet]. [cited 2022 Feb 14]. Available from: https://www.netzwerk-universitaetsmedizin.de/projekte/racoon

[7]   Salg GA, Ganten MK, Bucher AM, Kenngott HG, Fink MA, Seibold C, et al. A reporting and analysis framework for structured evaluation of COVID-19 clinical and imaging data. npj Digit Med. 2021 Apr 12;4(1):1-9. DOI: 10.1038/s41746-021-00439-y.

[8]   RACOON Network. RACOON Base – RACOON Infrastruktur [Internet]. [cited 2022 Feb 25]. Available from: https://racoon.network/?page_id=1638

[9]   Universitätsklinikum Frankfurt. Netzwerk Universitätsmedizin (NUM): Universitätsklinikum Frankfurt am Main [Internet]. [cited 2022 Feb 22]. Available from: https://www.kgu.de/ueber-uns/vorstand-des-universitaetsklinikums/aerztliche-direktion/stabsstelle-medizinische-informationssysteme-und-digitalisierung/netzwerk-universitaetsmedizin-num

[10]   Krefting D. Das Projekt CODEX des Netzwerks der Universitätsmedizin (NUM) [Internet]. 2021 [cited 2022 Feb 25]. Available from: https://www.miracum.org/wp-content/uploads/2021/07/2021_07_16_0930_Krefting_Das-Projekt-CODEX-des-Netzwerks-der-Universitaetsmedizin-NUM.pdf

[11]   Harris PA, Taylor R, Thielke R, Payne J, Gonzalez N, Conde JG. Research electronic data capture (REDCap)—A metadata-driven methodology and workflow process for providing translational research informatics support. Journal of Biomedical Informatics. 2009 Apr 1;42(2):377-381. DOI: 10.1016/j.jbi.2008.08.010.

[12]   Lautenschläger R, Kohlmayer F, Prasser F, Kuhn KA. A generic solution for web-based management of pseudonymized data. BMC Medical Informatics and Decision Making. 2015 Nov 30;15(1):100. DOI: 10.1186/s12911-015-0222-y.

[13]   Clinical Data Interchange Standards Consortium. ODM-XML | CDISC [Internet]. [cited 2022 Feb 25]. Available from: https://www.cdisc.org/standards/data-exchange/odm

[14]   Erbelding C, Sailer B, Stenzhorn H, Biergans S, Kohlmayer F, Kobak EM, et al. GECCO on FHIR – Towards Interoperable Data on COVID-19. In German Medical Science GMS Publishing House; 2021. p. DocAbstr. 38. DOI: 10.3205/21gmds012.

[15]   HL7 International. HL7 FHIR [Internet]. [cited 2022 Feb 27]. Available from: https://www.hl7.org/fhir/

[16]   Kapsner LA, Kampf MO, Seuchter SA, Gruendner J, Gulden C, Mate S, et al. Reduced Rate of Inpatient Hospital Admissions in 18 German University Hospitals During the COVID-19 Lockdown. Frontiers in Public Health. 2021;8. DOI: 10.3389/fpubh.2020.594117.

German Medical Data Sciences 2022 - Future Medicine
R. Röhrig et al. (Eds.)
© 2022 The authors and IOS Press.

doi:10.3233/SHTI220805

GRASCCO — The First Publicly Shareable, Multiply-Alienated German Clinical Text Corpus

Luise MODERSOHN [a,c,d,e*], Stefan SCHULZ [b,1*], Christina LOHR [a,d], and Udo HAHN [a,d]

[a] *JULIE Lab, Friedrich Schiller University Jena, Germany*
[b] *Institute for Medical Informatics, Statistics and Documentation, Medical University of Graz, Austria*
[c] *Intelligence and Informatics in Medicine, Medical Center rechts der Isar, Technical University Munich, Germany*
[d] *SMITH Consortium of the German Medical Informatics Initiative*
[e] *DIFUTURE Consortium of the German Medical Informatics Initiative*

Abstract. We describe the creation of GRASCCo, a novel German-language corpus composed of some 60 clinical documents with more than.43,000 tokens. GRASCCo is a synthetic corpus resulting from a series of alienation steps to obfuscate privacy-sensitive information contained in real clinical documents, the true origin of all GRASCCo texts. Therefore, it is publicly shareable without any legal restrictions We also explore whether this corpus still represents common clinical language use by comparison with a real (non-shareable) clinical corpus we developed as a contribution to the Medical Informatics Initiative in Germany (MII) within the SMITH consortium. We find evidence that such a claim can indeed be made.

Keywords. Clinical NLP, German Clinical Document Corpus, Case Reports

1. Introduction

Clinical natural language processing (cNLP) systematically suffers from a tremendous shortage of textual (meta-)data that can be used for training and evaluating NLP systems. This lack of data is mainly due to ethically motivated privacy concerns implemented by data protection legislation. The regulations derived therefrom interdict data/document sharing across different clinical sites and, even more so, with non-clinical, e.g., NLP, research groups – even after careful de-identification of privacy-sensitive information contained in clinical documents. This situation is particularly frustrating since sharing data and using shared data in competitively organized shared tasks are considered the main drivers of progress in the field of (biomedical) NLP [1,2].

As far as the German cNLP community is concerned, several clinical corpora have been created already, yet they are only accessible by local data management personnel on-site (for a survey, cf. [3]). Quite recently, the BRONCO150 corpus [4] has been set

---

[1] Corresponding author, Stefan Schulz, Medical University of Graz, Auenbruggerplatz 2, 8036 Graz, Austria, Email: Stefan.schulz@medunigraz.at
[*] These authors contributed equally to this work

up, which contains de-identified real clinical documents and is accessible upon demand via a Data Use Agreement (DUA). Clearly a milestone for German-language cNLP, this corpus also has some drawbacks: it is small in size (150 documents, 85,000 tokens) and its sentences have been shuffled randomly (to further increase data protection), which completely destroys the typical clinical document structure, e.g., in terms of sectioning. This destructive intervention not only affects medical plausibility but also dissolves any sort of inter-sentential referential relations, which is likely to negatively affect named entity recognition and relation extraction for language models trained on BRONCO.

With the exception of BRONCO150, no other German-language corpus made of *real* clinical documents is currently available for sharing. As an alternative, several research groups are considering the use of *synthetic* data resources, which simulate real clinical documents either by in-depth textual modifications of original clinical documents or by re-writing them from scratch. In the modification scenario, real clinical documents are the starting point for several rounds of alienation by experienced clinical experts, which include all kinds of paraphrasing, chopping and adding medical statements, changes of medical attributes, values, and other textual parameters relevant for re-identification attempts. All these changes, however, have to mimic the specific style and wording of the chosen report genre. The JSYNCC corpus [5] is a typical example of such a synthetic approach. It has been extracted from a wide range of introductory textbooks (e-books) for medical students. Obviously, this corpus cannot be distributed physically due to Intellectual Property Rights (IPRs), but JULIE Lab distributes the code to reliably re-create JSYNCC copies at any other physical site (including selected meta-data). As a prerequisite, all e-books incorporated in JSYNCC need to be licensed by the local institution. As another alternative, corpora have been developed, which are supposed to be *similar* in style and wording to real clinical documents. For instance, GGPONC [3] is a corpus composed of all German clinical guidelines for oncology and might be used as a proxy for real clinical data, if the degree of similarity is considered sufficient.

However, both synthetic and similar documents have to be examined how comparable they are to real clinical documents. Hence, in this paper, we not only describe the construction of a new synthetic German-language clinical corpus in Section 2, but also provide metrical evidence in Section 3 for its comparability to real (non-distributable) clinical documents. The latter are provided by the 3000PA corpus [6], a collection of more than 1,000 clinical documents each from the University Hospital of Jena (3000PAJ), Leipzig (3000PAL) and Aachen (3000PAA), respectively. Table 1 briefly summarizes major characteristics and attributes of the corpora relevant for this work.

Table 1 Overview of the German clinical text corpora

Corpus	Text Genre	# Documents	# Sentences	# Tokens	Shareability
3000PAJ [6]	Discharge summaries	1,106	146,191	1,707,019	Non-Shareable
JSYNCC OP [5]	Medical text-books	399	20,860	199,569	Code for re-creation
GGPONC 1.0 [3]	Clinical practice guidelines	12,761	77,986	1.522,588	DUA
BRONCO150 [4]	Discharge summaries	150	10,251	83,633	DUA
This work	**Alienated case reports**	**63**	**5,430**	**43.667**	**Fully Shareable**

2. Methods

The starting point for building the first version of GᴿᴀSCCᴏ (Graz Synthetic Clinical Corpus) was a heterogeneous collection of documents, to which the second first author (a medical doctor) had access for specific use in particular projects:

- Anonymized and pseudonymized discharge summaries from the University Hospital Freiburg, Germany,
- Anonymized and pseudonymized discharge summaries from KAGes, a large Austrian network of public hospitals,
- German case reports from Open Access journals,
- Discharge summaries, some of them not de-identified, published on the Web.

These documents cannot be shared as-is according to privacy regulations. In order to make them fully shareable, any references to real patients and clinical actors had to be removed. This led to a fictional re-creation of these reports (by the second first author). The transformations involved the following steps:

- Real names of patients and therapists were replaced by fictional names, often with gender assignments differing from the original documents,
- Completely fictitious place and institution names were added,
- All dates were placed in the future,
- To additionally increase the noise level for re-identification attacks, at least one factual change was introduced in each medically relevant sentence, e.g., concerning laboratory tests, test result values, patients' complaints, diagnoses, medication statements,
- Many passages were paraphrased at all linguistic levels (mostly lexically and syntactically),
- Text fragments were exchanged with other ones (flowing back and forth within the entire collection), especially when atypical medical phenomena were described.

In a second round, additional text alienations were carried out and regionally typical expressions for salutations, technical terms, abbreviations, and academic degrees were changed so that no conclusions about the true origin of the texts can be made.

The strong alienation in form and content of the synthesized documents entailed that some of these narratives became medically implausible. This is not an issue for NLP purposes, since their focus is on learning language (use) models rather than domain models. Once a document was considered safe from re-identifying all of the mentioned human individuals, according to the second first author's judgement, it was incorporated into the corpus. The entire collection was then published by the second first author as products of fiction "inspired by real clinic texts", and made publicly available under the Creative Commons license BY 4.0 (all rights attribution) at Zenodo.[2]

---

[2] https://zenodo.org/

3. Corpus Description and Comparison

We will now, first, give a detailed description of the synthetic GRaSCCo corpus (version 1), and then render preliminary evidence for its validity as a substitute for real clinical data by measuring the linguistic closeness between both document sets.

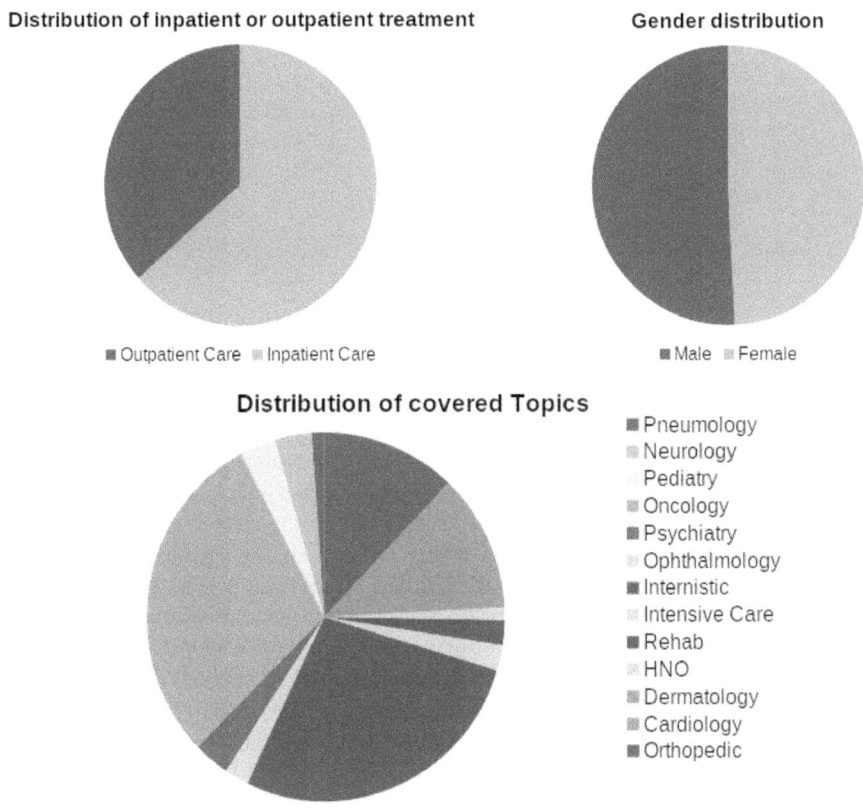

Figure 1. Document types, gender and topic distribution

GRaSCCo v.1 consists of 63 documents with about 5,000 sentences and 43,000 tokens. An average document comprises 93 sentences, with about 740 tokens. A more detailed quantitative comparison with alternative German medical datasets is depicted in Table 1. Our corpus is almost perfectly gender-balanced, covers two-thirds of all patients as hospitalized in-patients, and also incorporates a large variety of medical topics, such as ophthalmology, oncology, or orthopedics as visualized in Figure 1.

In order to judge whether the documents from GRaSCCo v.1 are truly linguistically close to real clinical documents, we took syntactic and semantic criteria into account and compared synthetic and real clinical corpora with non-clinical ones on a larger scale (for similar diagnostics of clinical reports, cf. also [7,8]).

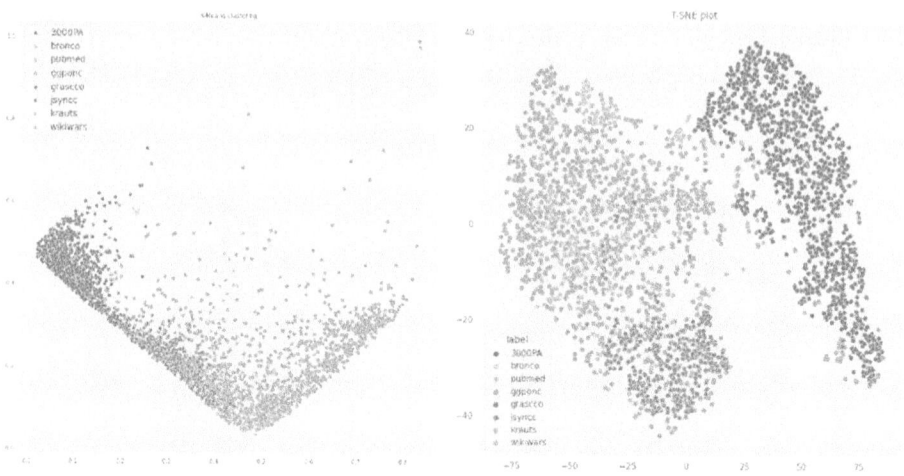

Figure 2. Clustering results of k-means (left) and t-SNE (right)

For syntactic measurements, we used SPACY[3] as a pipeline with the general German language model[4] to automatically count the number of sentences, tokens, stop words, nouns, verbs, etc. of each document (for a broader set of linguistic features, cf. [9]). As far as semantic criteria are concerned, we used a SPACY-based medical named entity extraction pipeline, with concepts from the Unified Medical Language System (UMLS) [10], such as Anatomy, Disorders or Living Being, and medication names from the ROTE LISTE.[5] The resulting normalized counts of sentences, tokens, and occurrences of named entities were used as features for the subsequent clustering step.

We used t-SNE (T-distributed Stochastic Neighbor Embedding) [11] and k-means to cluster the document features of our corpus and compared these aggregated data with those from other real clinical (the Jena part of 3000PA [6], BRONCO150 [4]), synthetic clinical (JSYNCC [5]), similar-to-clinical (GGPONC [3], German PUBMED case reports),[6] and non-clinical, i.e., Wikipedia- or newspaper-rooted German corpora (WIKIWARSDE [12] and KRAUTS [13]). This test was accomplished using the Python library *scikit-learn*[7] and its implementations of t-SNE and k-means.

We only used up to 1000 documents per dataset to ensure a more balanced and fair comparison. As can be seen from Figure 2, k-means clustering shows that all datasets are clearly distinguishable, albeit not perfectly separable. Thus, the selection of features seems to be appropriate to describe our datasets for comparison. Both the k-means and the t-SNE plot show a clear separation between the clinical 3000PA documents and the other ones. Interestingly, documents from GRASCCO v.1 can be found both in the

---

[3] https://spacy.io/
[4] *de_core_news_sm*: http://spacy.io/models/de
[5] https://www.rote-liste.de/produkte
[6] **Query:** Case Reports[Publication Type] AND GER[LA]
[7] https://scikit-learn.org/stable/index.html

3000PA and BRONCO150 cluster and near the JSYNCC cluster. This yields preliminary evidence that our synthetic corpus is, at least partially, comparable with real German discharge summaries.

4. Discussion

We introduced a new clinical German-language corpus, GRASCCO, which can be publicly distributed within the (c)NLP community without any legal or contractual constraints. We also assessed the linguistic closeness of this synthetic corpus to other clinical and non-clinical corpora. The results give first hints that GRASCCO might be a reasonable substitute for non-shareable real clinical corpora. With the unconstrained shareability and open usability of GRASCCO, we intend to contribute to better comparability of cNLP systems for the German language when GRASCCO is used as an experimental frame of reference.

GRASCCO is composed of synthetic documents, i.e., original, yet subsequently anonymized and content-wise altered, real German-language clinical documents. They have undergone several rounds of alienation so that the re-identification of individual patients can be ruled out to the best of our beliefs. A preliminary comparison with real German-language clinical documents reveals that they approximate these gold data at both the syntactic and semantic level of comparison. Thus, we may recommend GRASCCO as a reasonable, hopefully valid, substitute for real clinical documents, since the latter are out of reach for free distribution even after lots of additional curation efforts (e.g., trusted and certified de-identification). However, our comparison with real clinical data is currently limited in many ways. Both the syntactic and semantic features chosen for comparison are quite simplistic, the syntactic ones, in particular. We might easily complement simple sentence and token counts by more expressive features involving n-gram statistics or the syntactic complexity mirrored in parse trees (see [9] for additional, more sophisticated features). In a similar way, the comparison of overlapping medical terminology could also be complemented by incorporating lexical semantic relations, such as synonymy or taxonomies. However, these investigations are not the focus of this work but are under way using a stylistic workbench to be published elsewhere. Furthermore, providing semantic metadata (e.g., annotations for named entities and semantic relations holding between them) could be the starting point for establishing a commonly shared German-language clinical gold standard for training and evaluation in cNLP.

Follow-up versions of GRASCCO will contain more documents and further alienation steps to even more heavily perturb potential adverse attacks on these data. The corpus can be found under the following link:

DOI: https://doi.org/10.5281/zenodo.6539131

Declarations

Ethical vote: The usage of 3000PA (Jena) is based on the approval by the local ethics committee (4639-12/15) and the data protection officer of the Jena University Hospital.
Study-Registry: not applicable
Conflict of Interest: The authors declare that there is no conflict of interest.
Author contributions: StS: corpus design and data creation; LM: study design, LM, CL: data analysis and interpretation; LM, CL, StS, UH: paper writing, UH: manuscript coordination. All authors approved the manuscript in the submitted version and take responsibility for the scientific integrity of the work.
Acknowledgement: This work was supported by BMBF within the SMITH and DIFUTURE projects under grant 01ZZ1803G and 01ZZ2009, respectively. We thank André Scherag, Danny Ammon, and all members of the Data Integration Center of the Jena University Hospital for their continuous support.

References

[1] Huang CC, Lu Z. Community challenges in biomedical text mining over 10 years: success, failure and the future. Briefings in Bioinformatics. 2015;17(1):132-44. Available from: https://doi.org/10.1093/bib/bbv024.

[2] Nissim M, Abzianidze L, Evang K, van der Goot R, Haagsma H, Plank B, et al. Sharing is caring: the future of shared tasks. Computational Linguistics. 2017;43(4):897-904.

[3] Borchert F, Lohr C, Modersohn L, Langer T, Follmann M, Sachs JP, et al. GGPONC: a corpus of German medical text with rich metadata based on clinical practice guidelines. In: LOUHI 2020 – Proceedings of the 11th International Workshop on Health Text Mining and Information Analysis; 2020, pp. 38-48.

[4] Kittner M, Lamping M, Rieke DT, Götze J, Bajwa B, Jelas I, et al. Annotation and initial evaluation of a large annotated German oncological corpus. JAMIA Open. 2021;4(2). Ooab025. Available from: https://doi.org/10.1093/jamiaopen/ooab025.

[5] Lohr C, Buechel S, Hahn U. Sharing copies of synthetic clinical corpora without physical distribution: a case study to get around IPRs and privacy constraints featuring the German JSYNCC corpus. In: LREC 2018 – Proceedings of the 11th International Conference on Language Resources and Evaluation; 2018, pp. 1259-1266.

[6] Hahn U, Matthies F, Lohr C, Löffler M. 3000PA: towards a national reference corpus of German clinical language. In: Building Continents of Knowledge in Oceans of Data: The Future of Co-Created eHealth. vol. 247 of Studies in Health Technology and Informatics. IOS Press; 2018, pp. 26-30. Available from: https://doi.org/10.3233/978-1-61499-852-5-26.

[7] Campbell DA, Johnson SB. Comparing syntactic complexity in medical and non-medical corpora. In: AMIA 2001 – Proceedings of the 2001 Annual Symposium of the American Medical Informatics Association. A Medical Informatics Odyssey: Visions of the Future and Lessons from the Past; 2001, pp. 90-94.

[8] Lysanets Y, Morokhovets H, Bieliaieva, O. Stylistic features of case reports as a genre of medical discourse. Journal of Medical Case Reports. 2017; 11, #83.

[9] Neal T, Sundararajan K, Fatima A, Yan Y, Xiang Y, Woodard D. Surveying stylometry techniques and applications. ACM Computing Surveys. 2017;50(6):#86.

[10] Bodenreider O. The Unified Medical Language System (UMLS): integrating biomedical terminology. Nucleic Acids Research. 2004;32(suppl 1):D267-70. Available from: https://doi.org/10.1093/nar/gkh061.

[11] van der Maaten L, Hinton G. Visualizing data using t-SNE. Journal of Machine Learning Research. 2008;9(86):2579-605.

[12] Strötgen J, Gertz M. WikiWarsDE: a German corpus of narratives annotated with temporal expressions. In: Multilingual Resources and Multilingual Applications. GSCL 2011 – Proceedings of the Conference of the German Society for Computational Linguistics and Language Technology; 2011, pp. 129–134.

[13] Strötgen J, Minard AL, Lange L, Speranza M, Magnini B. KRAUTS: a German temporally annotated news corpus. In: LREC 2018 – Proceedings of the 11th International Conference on Language Resources and Evaluation. 2018, pp. 536-540.

German Medical Data Sciences 2022 - Future Medicine
R. Röhrig et al. (Eds.)
doi:10.3233/SHTI220806

Identifying Actionable Variants in Cancer - The Dual Web and Batch Processing Tool MTB -Report

Nadine S. KURZ[a,*], Júlia PERERA-BEL[b,*], Charlotte HÖLTERMANN[a], Tim
TUCHOLSKI[a], Jingyu YANG[a], Tim BEISSBARTH[a] and Jürgen DÖNITZ[a,1]

[a] *Dept. of Medical Bioinformatics, University Medical Center Göttingen, Germany*
[b] *MARGenomics, Hospital del Mar Medical Research Institute (IMIM), Spain*

Abstract. Next-generation sequencing methods continuously provide clinicians and
researchers in precision oncology with growing numbers of genomic variants found
in cancer. However, manually interpreting the list of variants to identify reliable
targets is an inefficient and cumbersome process that does not scale with the
increasing number of cases. Support by computer systems is needed for the analysis
of large scale experiments and clinical studies to identify new targets and therapies,
and user-friendly applications are needed in molecular tumor boards to support
clinicians in their decision-making processes. The MTB-Report tool annotates,
filters and sorts genetic variants with information from public databases, providing
evidence on actionable variants in both scenarios. A web interface supports medical
doctors in the tumor board, and a command line mode allows batch processing of
large datasets. The MTB-Report tool is available as an R implementation as well as
a Docker image to provide a tool that runs out-of-the-box. Moreover,
containerization ensures a stable application that delivers reproducible results over
time. A public version of the web interface is available at: http://mtb.bioinf.med.uni-
goettingen.de/mtb-report

Keywords. Variant interpretation, molecular tumor board, actionable variants,
molecular profiles, next-generation sequencing, precision oncology

1. Introduction

Next-generation sequencing (NGS) platforms are capable of generating large amounts
of clinically relevant data, especially in cancer genomics. The gained knowledge is being
deposited in a vast variety of databases and knowledge base resources [1], complicating
the task of gathering relevant information for clinicians and researchers alike.
Specifically the identification of actionable variants, i.e. genomic variants with relevance
for clinical decisions and cancer research, remains a challenge. Actionability in this
context may range from biomarkers for approved drugs following the indications of
cancer type, to cancer types not included in the drug indication (off-label use), or to
variants being studied in clinical trials.

The bioinformatician, pathologist or physician who obtained genomic data from a
patient tumor faces an overwhelming task. Having evaluated and filtered the data in

---

[1] Corresponding Author, Jürgen Dönitz, University Medical Center Göttingen (UMG), Goldschmidtstr.
1, 37077 Göttingen, Germany; E-mail: juergen.doenitz@bioinf.med.uni-goettingen de. * equal contribution.

terms of quality, the identified genomic variants need to be interrogated for biological and clinical implications. Mutations with well-established biological impact can be identified by accessing public knowledge sources (e.g. dbSNP [2], COSMIC [3], TCGA [4]) or by applying prediction models (e.g. SIFT [5], PolyPhen-2 [6], IntOGen [7]). A detailed overview of available data resources and tools for cancer variant interpretation is provided by [8].

However, in case the variant under investigation is not associated with clear clinical evidence (e.g. an ALK mutation or amplification instead of rearrangements, unknown BRAF mutation), a range of questions arises: is this mutation a loss or gain of function (LoF and GoF, respectively)? Does it confer sensitivity to any targeted drug? Is there any existing evidence on this variant in another cancer type? Does it result in resistance, or in susceptibility to certain treatments?

Many institutions are therefore making efforts to gather and structure information from clinical trials, case reports, publications of preclinical experimental research as well as guidelines and approval organizations in online databases. Among these essential efforts we find CIViC [9], GDKD [10], OncoKB [11], My Cancer Genome [12] and PMKB [13]. Yet, these resources are not aimed at querying multiple variants at a time, as is usually the case when a tumor genome is sequenced. Tools to interpret tumor genomes are arising, such as Cancer Genome Interpreter [14] and Personal Cancer Genome Reporter (PCGR) [15], however none of these tools offer the option to be run locally on large amounts of variant data, as is often needed in cancer research and bioinformatics.

Here, we present MTB-Report, an application that can be used on the one hand as a web interface aiming for the manual preparation of patient data for a molecular tumor board. On the other hand, it can be used as a command line tool to process large data sets to analyze data of wet lab experiments and large-scale screens. The tool is containerized as a Docker image which switches to one of these two modi based on the container runtime parameters.

2. Methods

2.1. Input data structure

The provided variants for MTB-Report may be Single Nucleotide Variants (SNVs), Copy Number Variants (CNVs) or fusion proteins. Input data can be uploaded in several tabular data formats (TXT, CSV, XLSX), yet they require a certain structure. SNVs are accepted as Variant Call Format (VCF), Mutation Annotation Format (MAF) files or as text files with a table with at least three columns (gene, variant type, variant). The genomic locations that are stored in VCF or MAF files are internally converted to protein locations, the typical variant format in public databases, in an automated fashion. CNVs must be a table with at least two columns: The first column contains gene symbols, the second column specifies the type of copy number alteration (amplification or deletion). Gene fusions must be a table with two columns, each contains one of the two affected genes of a fusion gene. For the gene names, the gene names defined by the HUGO Gene Nomenclature Committee [16] at the European Bioinformatics Institute should be used.

2.2. Databases

Genomic input data are queried against databases specialized on cancer predictive biomarkers. The user can select among the following databases:

- Gene Drug Knowledge Database - GDKD [10]: Expert-curated database that focuses exclusively on somatic variants which predict response to anti-cancer drugs (genomic predictive biomarkers). Variants with preclinical evidence are filtered based on their scientific soundness and translational power.
- Clinical Interpretation of Variants in Cancer - CIViC [9]: Expert-crowdsourced knowledgebase for the curation of genomic biomarkers in cancer: prognostic, diagnostic, predisposing and predictive. It also contains both germline and somatic variants.
- OnkoKB [11] is another database for precision medicine from the Memorial Sloan Kettering Cancer Center. For nearly 700 genes with around 5700 alterations are evidence-based information. Due to license limitations, the database is not distributed as part of the MTB-Report implementation, but can be provided by the user.
- Tumor Alterations Relevant for Genomics-driven Therapy - TARGET [17]: Consists of a list of 135 genes manually curated by experts from the Dana-Farber Cancer Institute with predictive, prognostic and diagnostic implications in cancer.
- Meric-Bernstam et al., 2015 [18]: List of therapeutically actionable genes (i.e. predictive biomarkers) with a focus on genes included as selection criteria in clinical trials.

By default, MTB-Report embeds the latest database versions. Apart from [11], the databases are included by default and can optionally be provided by the user in case a specific database version is required.

3. Results

The MTB-Report tool is a convenient tool which supports the two important use cases of precision oncology - supporting molecular tumor boards by providing actionable variants to clinicians as well as reporting actionability for large scale data analyses in cancer research. The underlying computational algorithm and methods have previously been published in [19], where an evaluation of the results showed very high sensitivity in the detection of actionable variants.

3.1. Code availability and portability

The application is available as an R implementation published as Open Source. Additionally, the implementation is available as a Docker image to provide a platform-independent environment for the application. The dependencies are conveniently shipped with the application, and thus ensure a stable tool out of the box and allow results to be reproducible. The Docker image can be used to start both the web server for interactive analysis or batch processing mode on the command line. A public instance of the web application is available at http://mtb.bioinf.med.uni-goettingen.de/mtb-report. The source code is available at https://gitlab.gwdg.de/MedBioinf/mtb/mtb-report.

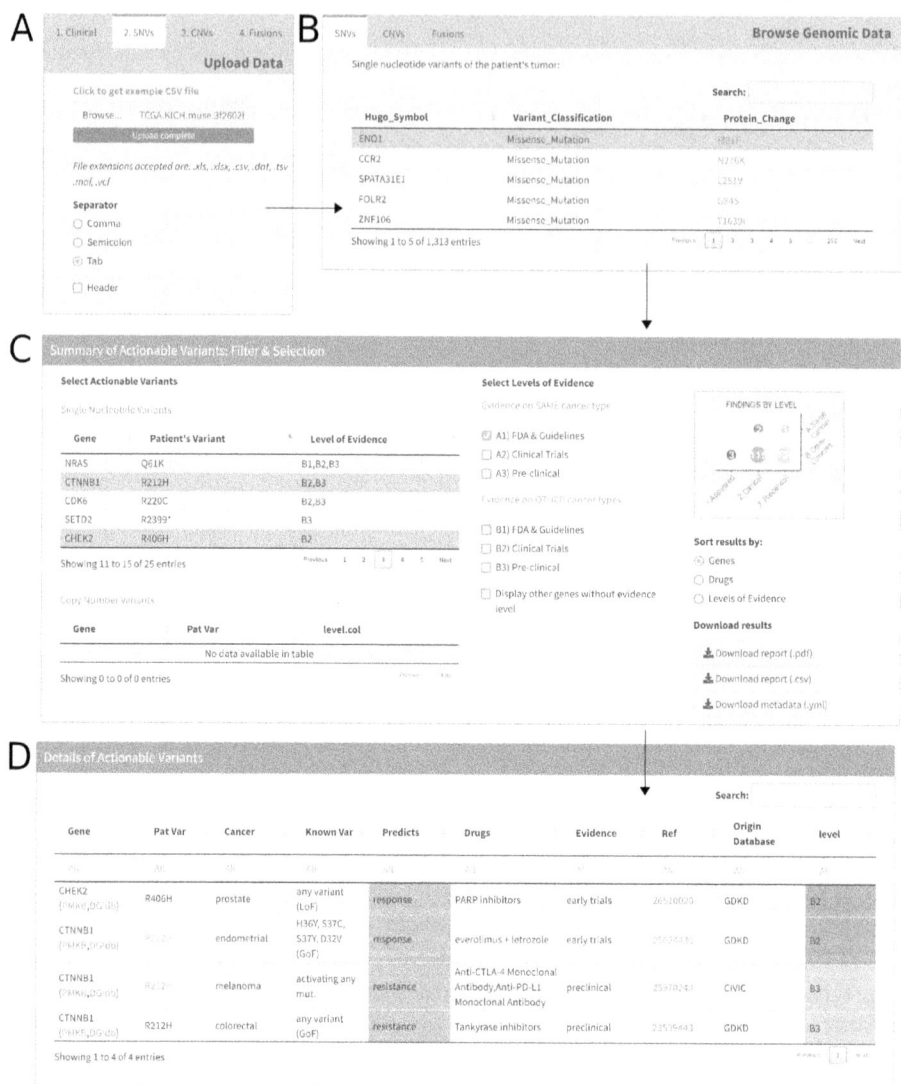

Figure 1. User interface of MTB-Report, showing A) the input form for patient data, B) a genome browser, and C) the results section of a query displaying the identified actionable variants. D) Upon selection of one or multiple variants, the details of all evidence linked to these variants are displayed in the table of results.

3.2. The web application

The interactive web application is written in R using the Shiny framework [20]. It is launched automatically by the Docker container when no input files are provided, and can then be accessed locally using a browser at http://localhost:3838/mtb-report. The graphical user interface (GUI) guides the user through several steps of data input, enabling a convenient environment for uploading genomic variants and adding metadata about the patient. Of note, this patient data is not used in querying the databases and thus does not influence the results, but is instead appended to the output tables to be used in subsequent analyses. The application does not apply quality filters to the variants provided: it assumes that the input only contains high quality variants. Additionally, the user can explore sample data from the TCGA [4] project.

After providing the variant and patient data in the input form, MTB-Report provides multiple possibilities to browse the parsed genomic data. In a first summary box ("Summary of Actionable Variants: Filter & Selection", Figure 1) the identified actionable variants are listed. This summary by variant displays the evidence level associated to that variant, and any genomic quality provided as input by the user. An additional summary by level of evidence is depicted in a figure (with the number of findings at each level). By selecting a variant or a level of evidence, the detailed information of the actionability of a variant is displayed in the box "Details of Actionable Variants" (Figure 1). The table can be filtered by selecting one or several variants and levels of evidence. If more than one selection is applied, the union of the selection is displayed. The results can be sorted by genes, by drugs or by levels of evidence (though the interactive table allows sorting by each column, the download option will retain this selection for the generated report file). The detailed table can further be sorted according to columns or searched for specific patterns. Links to important databases of clinical implications of genomic variants such as PMKB [13] and DGIdb [21] are provided. Furthermore, the user can verify the variant-drug association with the original source. A report in Portable Document Format (PDF) or Comma-separated values (CSV) format of these results can be downloaded, where actionable variants are sorted according to their relevance in the final report.

```
data:
    path: input.maf
        cancer_type: pancreas    # only for documentation
        variation_type: snv
        ref_genome: hg38    # only for documentation
    tool:
        git_checksum: aac6608c
        date: '2022-02-27'
    databases:
        gdkd: v20.0
        civic: 15-jan-01
        target_meric: v3
        oncokb: v1
```

Figure 2. Part of a sample metadata file generated by MTB-Report. The first section describes the input data, the following sections are generated by MTB-Report and define the software and databases' versions.

3.3. Batch processing

Providing the files to be analyzed as command line arguments, the MTB-Report results are processed without launching the GUI, returning the results in CSV-formatted tables. The reported actionability of queried variants is identical in the web and batch processing modes, however, the CSV output generated by the batch mode is more suitable for downstream analysis, and can be further processed. Additional information, corresponding to the patient and cancer type information that can be provided in the web version, may be provided by passing an optional metadata file in YAML format as a command line parameter. The metadata file can contain several sets of input files for different patients or different cell lines. This way, the simultaneous analysis of large-scale studies with multiple patients or biological model systems is possible.

The metadata file is not only used to structure the input, the MTB-Report tool also writes relevant information back into the YAML file. The data generated by MTB-Report includes all relevant information to make the results fully reproducible, including the MTB-Report version, the consulted databases and their versions as well as the input and output files. An example metadata file is partially listed in Figure 2.

4. Discussion

With MTB-Report we have implemented a tool for precision oncology, with an implementation of an R-based web application for the evidence-based reporting strategy for molecular tumor boards and a command line tool for large scale data projects. MTB-Report focuses on finding evidence-based actionable variants and provides an expanded catalog by reporting cancer type repurposing and low evidence levels. MTB-Report is available as a public domain tool and a stand-alone tool, a public instance is available on the institute's web page. In this way, it fits the needs of both clinicians who may use an up-to-date version of the web application, and bioinformaticians, who can install the application locally and integrate it in in-house-pipelines and custom analyses.

As the protection of sensitive patient data is one of the most important requirements in clinical deployments, all database files may be included based on the local host file system. MTB-Report can thus be installed in protected local area networks and is fully functional with restricted or no internet connections. Furthermore, the source code is freely available, which allows insights into the code and a custom local build of the Docker image.

More tools aim to provide web applications and tools for precision oncology, examples are cBioPortal [22], MTB Portal [23], the Cancer Genome Interpreter [14], PanDrugs [24], IMPACT [25,26] and MIRACUM-Pipe [27]. These tools are comparable to MTB-Report, as they focus on cancer variants, allowing a multi-query of genomic variants against selected databases and applying algorithms (heuristic or predictive) to prioritize drugs. With regard to approved drugs, all tools rely on the same resources. However, expanding the therapeutic landscape, each tool uses its own approach. For instance, the Cancer Genome Interpreter identifies driver mutations and uses the Catalog of Validated Oncogenic Mutations and the Cancer Biomarkers database [14], maintained by the same group, to identify actionable driver variants. The PCGR [15] performs multiple oncology-relevant annotations (CIViC [9], Cancer Biomarkers database [14], ClinVar [28], COSMIC [3], DGIdb [21], etc.) from VCF files. VCF files allow PCGR to include additional information retrieved from the genomic data (e.g. MSI status, mutational signatures, and mutational burden). The output is a tiered interactive report in Hypertext Markup Language (HTML) format that is intended for clinical translation. PanDrugs [24] integrates multiple resources and provides a curated model for drug annotations. This tool puts emphasis on indirect targeting and pathway repurposing, and ranks drugs according to a weighted model that considers the number of alterations supporting evidence for a drug. The IMPACT pipeline [25,26] and web portal have a strong focus on pharmacogenomic (drug-target) interactions and rank drugs as well, by computing a hypergeometric test that considers the number of alterations supporting evidence for a drug. The advantage of MTB-Report is its dual use feature to use the same methods for single patients and large-scale data projects.

All these examples show the variability between reporting tools with regard to the databases used, the prioritization rules, and the visualization approaches. It is important to note that MTB-Report is a reporting tool, and, as such, does not provide any treatment suggestions and leaves the decision to the liable person. It serves as a tool to compile and visualize available information for the treating physicians or researchers. The quality of the displayed information is therefore heavily dependent on the quality of the provided databases. In contrast, so-called treatment algorithms incorporate expert rules into the NGS bioinformatic pipeline with the final aim of assigning a treatment to a patient. Treatment algorithms ensure standardization and reproducibility by regulating technical aspects of data processing such as minimum coverage, allele frequency, fold change, size of amplicons, prediction scores, as well as the rules to match variants to drug prescription. Hence, treatment algorithms are suitable for clinical trials. The methods presented here and in [19] are still under development and for research purpose only.

5. Declarations

Ethical vote: Not applicable

Conflict of interest: The authors declare that they have no competing interests.

Authors contributions: JPB, TB: design and concept of the application and user interface; CH, JD: concept of the batch processing; NSK, JPB, CH, TT, JY: R software implementation; NSK, JPB, CH, JD, TB writing the manuscript; All authors approved the manuscript in the submitted version and take responsibility for the scientific integrity of the work.

Funding: This work was supported by the Volkswagen Foundation within research project MTB-Report (ZN3424) and by the German Ministry of Education and Research (BMBF) projects Genoperspektiv [01GP1402], MyPathSem [031L0024], HER2LOW [031A429] and MMML-Demonstrators [031A428].

References

[1] Good BM, Ainscough BJ, McMichael JF, Su AI, Griffith OL. Organizing knowledge to enable personalization of medicine in cancer. Genome Biol. 2014 Aug 27;15(8):438, doi: 10.1186/s13059-014-0438-7.

[2] Sherry ST, Ward MH, Kholodov M, Baker J, Phan L, Smigielski EM, et al. dbSNP: the NCBI database of genetic variation. Nucleic Acids Res. 2001 Jan 1;29(1):308–11, doi:10.1093/nar/29.1.308.

[3] Forbes SA, Beare D, Boutselakis H, Bamford S, Bindal N, Tate J, et al. COSMIC: somatic cancer genetics at high-resolution. Nucleic Acids Res. 2017 Jan 4;45(D1):D777–83, doi: 10.1093/nar/gkw1121.

[4] Weinstein JN, Collisson EA, Mills GB, Shaw KM, Ozenberger BA, Ellrott K, et al. The Cancer Genome Atlas Pan-Cancer Analysis Project. Nat Genet. 2013 Oct;45(10):1113–20, doi: 10.1038/ng.2764.

[5] Ng PC, Henikoff S. SIFT: Predicting amino acid changes that affect protein function. Nucleic Acids Res. 2003 Jul 1;31(13):3812-4, doi: 10.1093/nar/gkg509.

[6] Adzhubei IA, Schmidt S, Peshkin L, Ramensky VE, Gerasimova A, Bork P, et al. A method and server for predicting damaging missense mutations. Nat Methods. 2010 Apr,7(4):248-9, doi: 10.1002/0471142905.hg0720s76.

[7] Gonzalez-Perez A, Perez-Llamas C, Deu-Pons J, Tamborero D, Schroeder MP, Jene-Sanz A, et al. IntOGen-mutations identifies cancer drivers across tumor types. Nat Methods. 2013 Nov;10(11):1081-2, doi: 10.1038/nmeth.2642.

[8]   Borchert F, Mock A, Tomczak A., Hügel J, Alkarkoukly S, Knurr A, et al. Knowledge bases and software support for variant interpretation in precision oncology. Brief Bioinform. 2021 Nov 5;22(6), doi:10.1093/bib/bbab134.

[9]   Griffith M, Spies NC, Krysiak K, McMichael JF, Coffman AC, Danos AM, et al. CIViC is a community knowledgebase for expert crowdsourcing the clinical interpretation of variants in cancer. Nat Genet. 2017 Feb;49(2):170–4, doi: 10.1038/ng.3774.

[10]   Dienstmann R, Jang IS, Bot B, Friend S, Guinney J. Database of genomic biomarkers for cancer drugs and clinical targetability in solid tumors. Cancer Discov. 2015 Feb 1;5(2):118–23, doi: 10.1158/2159-8290.CD-14-1118.

[11]   Chakravarty D, Gao J, Phillips S, Kundra R, Zhang H, Wang J, et al. OncoKB: A Precision Oncology Knowledge Base. JCO Precision Oncology. 2017 May 16;(1):1–16, doi: 10.1200/PO.17.00011.

[12]   Holt ME, Mittendorf KF, LeNoue-Newton M, Jain NM, Anderson I, Lovly CM, et al. My Cancer Genome: Coevolution of precision oncology and a molecular oncology knowledgebase. JCO Clinical Cancer Informatics. 2021 Dec;(5):995-1004, doi: 10.1200/CCI.21.00084.

[13]   Huang L, Fernandes H, Zia H, Tavassoli P, Rennert H, Pisapia D, et al. The cancer precision medicine knowledge base for structured clinical-grade mutations and interpretations. J Am Med Inform Assoc. 2017 May 1;24(3):513–9, doi: 10.1093/jamia/ocw148.

[14]   Tamborero D, Rubio-Perez C, Deu-Pons J, Schroeder MP, Vivancos A, Rovira A, et al. Cancer Genome Interpreter annotates the biological and clinical relevance of tumor alterations. Genome Medicine. 2018 Mar 28;10(1):25, doi: 10.1186/s13073-018-0531-8.

[15]   Nakken S, Fournous G, Vodák D, Aasheim LB, Myklebost O, Hovig E. Personal Cancer Genome Reporter: variant interpretation report for precision oncology. Bioinformatics. 2018; 34(10), 1778-1780, doi: 10.1093/bioinformatics/btx817.

[16]   Povey S, Lovering R, Bruford E, Wright M, Lush M, Wain H. The HUGO gene nomenclature committee (HGNC). Hum Genet. 2001 Dec;109(6):678-80, doi: 10.1007/s00439-001-0615-0.

[17]   Van Allen EM, Wagle N, Stojanov P, Perrin DL, Cibulskis K, Marlow S, et al. Whole-exome sequencing and clinical interpretation of formalin-fixed, paraffin-embedded tumor samples to guide precision cancer medicine. Nat Med. 2014 Jun;20(6):682-8, doi: 10.1038/nm.3559.

[18]   Meric-Bernstam F, Johnson A, Holla V, Bailey AM, Brusco L, Chen K, et al. A decision support framework for genomically informed investigational cancer therapy. J Natl Cancer Inst. 2015 Jul;107(7), doi: 10.1093/jnci/djv098.

[19]   Perera-Bel J, Hutter B, Heining C, Bleckmann A, Fröhlich M, Fröhling S, et al. From somatic variants towards precision oncology: Evidence-driven reporting of treatment options in molecular tumor boards. Genome Med. 2018; 10(1), 1-15, doi: 10.1186/s13073-018-0529-2.

[20]   Chang W, Cheng J, Allaire JJ, Sievert C, Schloerke B, Xie Y, Allen J, McPherson J, Dipert A, Borges B. shiny: Web Application Framework for R [Internet]. 201821. Available from: https://CRAN.R-project.org/package=shiny

[21]   Griffith M, Griffith OL, Coffman AC, Weible JV, McMichael JF, Spies NC, et al. DGIdb: mining the druggable genome. Nat Methods. 2013 Dec;10(12):1209–10, doi: 10.1038/nmeth.2689.

[22]   Gao, J, Aksoy, BA, Dogrusoz, U, Dresdner, G, Gross, B, Sumer, SO, et al. Integrative analysis of complex cancer genomics and clinical profiles using the cBioPortal. Science signaling. 2013 Apr 2;6(269):pl1-pl1, doi: 10.1126/scisignal.2004088.

[23]   Tamborero D, Dienstmann R, Rachid MH, Boekel J, Lopez-Fernandez A, Jonsson M et al. The Molecular Tumor Board Portal supports clinical decisions and automated reporting for precision oncology. Nat Cancer. 2022 Feb;3(2):251-61, doi: 10.1038/s43018-022-00332-x.

[24]   Piñeiro-Yáñez E, Reboiro-Jato M, Gómez-López G, Perales-Patón J, Troulé K, Rodríguez JM, et al. PanDrugs: a novel method to prioritize anticancer drug treatments according to individual genomic data. Genome Med. 2018 May 31;10(1):41, doi:10.1186/s13073-018-0546-1.

[25]   Hintzsche J, Kim J, Yadav V, Amato C, Robinson SE, Seelenfreund E, et al. IMPACT: a whole-exome sequencing analysis pipeline for integrating molecular profiles with actionable therapeutics in clinical samples. J Am Med Inform Assoc. 2016 Jul;23(4):721-30, doi:10.1093/jamia/ocw022.

[26]   Hintzsche JD, Yoo M, Kim J, Amato CM, Robinson WA, Tan AC. IMPACT web portal: oncology database integrating molecular profiles with actionable therapeutics. BMC Medical Genomics. 2018 Apr 20;11(2):26, doi: 10.1186/s12920-018-0350-1.

[27]   Metzger P, Scheible R, Hess M, et al. Miracum-Pipe. https://github.com/AG-Boerries/MIRACUM-Pipe (10 May 2022, date last accessed).

[28]   Landrum MJ, Lee JM, Riley GR, Jang W, Rubinstein WS, Church DM, et al. ClinVar: public archive of relationships among sequence variation and human phenotype. Nucleic Acids Res. 2014 Jan;42(D1):D980-985, doi: 10.1093/nar/gkt1113.

German Medical Data Sciences 2022 - Future Medicine
R. Röhrig et al. (Eds.)
doi:10.3233/SHTI220807

What Went Wrong in eMedCare? Formative Evaluation of an IT Project in Primary Care in Two Rural Districts

Mareike PRZYSUCHA[a], Lara PETERS[b], Andreas BÜSCHER[b], Martin
SCHNELLHAMMER[c], Ursula HÜBNER[a1]

[a] Health Informatics Research Group, Osnabrück University of AS, Germany
[b] Nursing Science, Osnabrück University of AS, Germany
[c] Living Lab, Osnabrück University of AS, Germany

Abstract. Introduction The interaction between nurses and physicians in the primary care setting is challenging with regard to structural, process and technical barriers. In order to overcome these barriers, the eMedCare project was launched and a commercial system was implemented. **Objective** This study aimed at a formative evaluation of the project. The findings should be used retrospectively to understand the failure of the project. **Methods** To this end, two rounds of qualitative interviews with 10 respectively 8 healthcare providers were performed. **Results** The interviews revealed a mixed benefit. Difficulties arose because the initial aim to monitor patients shifted towards improving the communication between the providers, partly due to the poor usability of the monitoring system. Additional workload was imposed because the system was not interoperable with the institutional IT systems. **Conclusion** Projects with an unclear or shifting vision and focus seem to be susceptible to failure. The secure communication applications could have been realised on the intended scale if the national *Telematikinfrastruktur* had been in place.

Keywords. Primary care, physicians, nurses, patient monitoring, provider communication

1. Introduction

The provision of care across professions and organizations is challenging with respect to continuity of care [1] which is generally true, however particularly when the professionals are scattered over practices and facilities such as it is the case in the primary care setting. Health IT systems, e. g. to support communication, are a means to mitigate these challenges by supporting information continuity, one of the dimensions of continuity of care [1]. Despite its great potential, the use of health IT systems does not remedy these problems alone, in particular as details about the type of cooperation have to be settled before health IT can unfold its power [2]. Furthermore, there are still barriers even once the cooperation has been established which can be broken down into structural,

---

[1] Corresponding Author: Ursula H. Hübner, Hochschule Osnabrück, Health Informatics Research Group, D-49009 Osnabrück, Germany; E-mail: u.huebner@hs-osnabrueck.de.

ideological, organisational and relational barriers [3–5]. In addition, health IT can be a barrier in itself, e.g. when usability is compromised [6].

While all these barriers are well known and are – in principle – avoidable, there are many projects that do not succeed in supporting to establish information continuity. This paper will therefore take the perspective of a failed project and summarise the lessons learned. The paper is based on a study that aimed to evaluate the use of a health IT system for physicians and nurses in primary care. This formative evaluation should focus on the users' perception of the IT system's impact on the care delivery processes and on the identification of use cases that were well and less well covered by the IT system.

2. Methods

2.1. Organisational Settings

The study was embedded into the project eMedCare, conducted by two rural districts in Western Lower Saxony, Germany, of whom one initiated and financially managed the project. After the project funding was granted, a call for tenders was published for the IT system of the project, to which only one vendor responded who then was selected.

In the project, three nursing care facilities (two nursing homes and one home-care service) and four practices of general practitioners (GPs) agreed to cooperate in order to improve the care of their patients by allowing a more continuous monitoring of physiological parameters, such as vital signs, blood glucose level and ECG. Each nursing care facility worked at least with one practice. For each pair of practice – nursing care facility, only patients (n = 28) were included who themselves or their guardians consented to participate.

2.2. System description and system in use

In order to perform the measurements at the point of care an off-the-shelf commercial system was implemented. All devices necessary to measure weight, blood pressure, glucose, pulse, oxygen saturation, peak flow, temperature, heart activity (via ECG) were included in a backpack. These devices could be operated by a tablet computer. Depending on the role of the user, the software on the tablet offered different functions. Physicians were able to order measurements and questionnaires and view the results, nurses could view these orders, perform measurements using the devices from the backpack or enter the measurements manually, and send these data. Nurses were also able to enter information provided by the patients into a questionnaire. While the nurses used the system mainly via the tablet, the physicians requested the measurements/ questionnaire data and viewed the findings typically via a web portal. This web portal also included an alarm function for the physicians which could be calibrated individually for each patient, and different modes of data visualisation. Patients had no direct access to their data in this phase of the project. A general overview of the IT-system is shown in Figure 1.

All three nursing care facilities already used IT systems. Two of them used MediFox Dan, which by that time only included an interface for financial data, but also provided access for physicians [7]. The last nursing care facility used a product from DM EDV, which by that time provided interfaces to applications within the MS suite and for financial data [8].

To evaluate the IT system formatively, two rounds of guided expert interviews were conducted. In the first round (June to August 2019), five general practitioners and five nurses (two from a home care service; three from a nursing home) participated. Two nurses worked as nursing managers while the remaining three had an executive function. Out of all ten participants, there were five males and five females. Focusing on the general setting, ten open-ended questions of the interviews served to reveal the perceived impact of the eMedCare IT system on the care processes. In the second round (February to August 2020 – delays due to Covid-19), four general practitioners and three nurses (one from a home care service, two from nursing homes) were interviewed. In total three males und four females participated. All of them had taken part in the first round as well. Here, the interviews focused on identifying use cases and scenarios which were well or less well supported by the system.

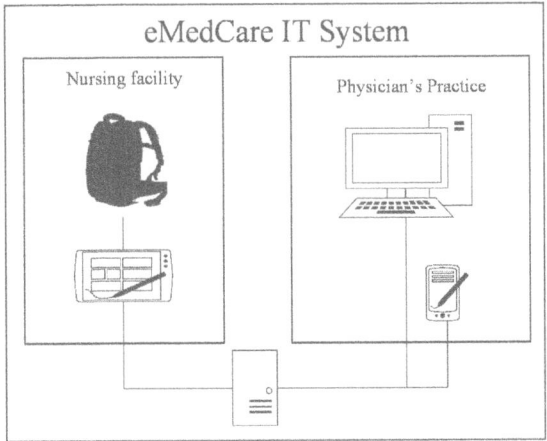

Figure 1. Overview of the final IT system structure used in eMedCare

During both phases, each facility was represented by at least one participant. The interviews in both rounds were audio recorded, transcribed and the transcripts analysed according to qualitative content analysis [9]. The transcripts of the second round were furthermore translated into UML use case, process and class diagrams using Visual Paradigm V16 to identify well and poorly supported processes.

It is noteworthy, that major software changes were realised between the first and second round due to the feedback giving in round one. These changes included new features such as a chat that was added to the application on the tablets together with a chat app for the physicians, and a function for taking and submitting annotated photos was integrated as well as the opportunity to submit documents like requests for prescriptions.

After interview round two was finished the project came to an end and the application was abandoned.

3. Results

3.1. Round one: New processes, more workload, mixed benefit

Impact on health care provision

The healthcare providers noted some benefits. In particular, the GPs reported that the IT system could be used as a tool to prepare visits, and the digital patient record allowed nurses in the home care setting to access data even though they were not at the patient's home. However, there were also major difficulties recognised by the healthcare providers. They complained about a higher workload due to the IT system. The general practitioners stated that they actively needed to look into the portal to find out whether there were new data. Nurses told that they had extra tasks to fulfil. These tasks also led to more documentation as double or triple documentation was necessary due to lacking interfaces between the devices and the institutional IT systems. The participants also reported that the access to data improved, but in some cases the number of direct contacts between the physicians and their patients decreased. Another point referred to the usefulness of devices from the backpack. The nurses did not regard them as very functional.

Impact on teamwork, communication, and cooperation

The participants stated that the cooperation as such was not influenced. Although the data were transmitted immediately at the point of care, they were not read by the physicians once they came in. Consequently, they feared to oversee information. Thus, they preferred communication via fax. The nurses stated that the IT-system still required to reach out to a physician via phone and this took time. Recalls from physicians then often reached the next shift, who were not familiar with the reason for the call.

The project itself

Participants reported that it took some time to adapt to the changing processes. Some also reported that the workload increased due to the new processes imposed by the project. A physician remarked that the number of tasks should not be too large and the frequency of measurements not too high to avoid time pressure on nurses.

Outlook

Due to the limited number of health care organizations included and the small number of patients included into the project, the participants stated that in inclusion of other disciplines and professions and the inclusion of more patients might lead to more communication and therefore to a higher impact. The participants also wished to shift from a system mainly for documentation and monitoring to a system that supported the communication (including video calls) between the healthcare providers. They also proposed to integrate the national medication record ("Medikationsplan").

3.2. Round two: Shift of focus

During the second round of the formative evaluation, it became clear that the project focus had shifted from realising an application for monitoring and documentation towards an application for communication. The chat app for smartphones was made available that the users had requested.

Usage of IT

Out of all functions offered by the IT system at the interview round two, the chat and the photo function were the ones that were predominantly used. Other functions – in particular for measuring vital signs and other physiological parameters – were hardly used, except of measuring the blood glucose level. One reason for not using these monitoring functions was that the devices were still (like in round one) not considered to be suitable for this purpose. For example, the scale was described as too small. Furthermore, it was stated that patients with dementia pulled off the ECG electrodes before all electrodes could be applied and the measurements could start. Another factor was that the backpack was found to be too big, heavy and bulky for female nurses in home care. An overview of use cases available, not used and desirable is given in Table 1. It shows that beyond the measurement functions and the communication functions further applications were found to be desirable but not available in the eMedCare system.

Table 1: Use cases available, not used and desirable

Use Case	Currently available	Available but not used	Desirable but not available
Ordering measurements and other tasks (physician -> nurse)	x		
Measuring vital signs and other physiological parameters		x	
Integrating tasks and measurement data in institutional IT-system			x
Documentation: wound assessment including photo documentation	x		
Chats: writing, reading	x		
eMail / chat: sharing documents			x
ePrescription: medication			x
Medication record: sharing, reading ("*Medikationsplan*")			x
ePrescription: ordering nursing care at home "Häusliche Krankenpflege"			x

Impact on teamwork, communication, and cooperation

Due to the integrated chat, the communication between facilities was improved. Instead of calling a practice several times and waiting for someone to respond to the call, asking the physician for an answer and calling back to reply to a question, the nurses used the chat function to write their question and the physician could answer. Only in case of an emergency, the nurses called the practice or directly the ambulance.

The project itself

Within the project each nursing care facility cooperated with one or two practices, though they had patients from different general practitioners. Also, each general practitioner cooperated with only one nursing care facility within the project, though they might have patients in other nursing settings as well. Out of this small number of patients, not all participated in the project. This led to a very small number of patients being included into the project. Therefore, the participants always used the "normal" way to communicate, the communication via eMedCare came on top. For each patient, the participants had to look whether they were part of the eMedCare project. Thus, a nursing care facility and a practice might have to use eMedCare for patient A and the "normal" communication for patient B.

One participant did not see the need to change communication ways as the current ways were rated as sufficient. However, a missing commitment to communicate via the new chat function was also criticised and an obligation to do so was demanded.

Outlook

In addition to the outlook of round one, participants wished for a reproduction of the whole prescription process (request for a prescription, medication record, ePrescription) within the IT system in order to improve their workflow.

4. Discussion

Although the nurses and physicians recognised some benefits of the eMedCare IT system, the functions provided did not match the expectations overall. Due to usability and interoperability issues, the integration into the workflows was poor. The nurses performed extra tasks in addition to the already high workload. Furthermore, the eMedCare system as a monitoring turned out to be only partly useful and functional. On top of this, the focus of the users shifted during the use towards a communication application. All these deficits emerged during the course of the project, because there was no real agreement to change the collaboration and communication processes - for the few patients in this project and for a larger number in the future.

Even though the number of patients was a barrier, some of the problems which arose during the project, would also have come up with more patients. The lacking interfaces between devices and IT systems would still have led to a higher documentation burden. Many of the perceived difficulties arose from a lack of pertinent applications within the national IT infrastructure for health care (*Telematikinfrastruktur*), such as a national electronic health records, secure communication systems like e-mail and chat, and applications for medication processes, as well as the missing obligation to provide interoperable systems. Whether these services will become available as promised [10] remains to be seen.

In the end, the project members abandoned the eMedCare system after the project had finished. They did not request the two districts to continue or to extend the project. Abandonment is a phenomenon rather neglected in research but seen in practice and addressed by the NASSS framework that brings together issues of non-adoption, abandonment, scale-up, spread, and sustainability (NASSS) [11]. The authors of the NASSS framework contend that complicated scenarios tend to be prone to abandonment. Most strikingly were the following criteria that match the statements of the users in eMedCare (Table 2).

The findings from this project have to be regarded as an illustration of how projects can fail. They do not claim to be representative and the generalisation is therefore limited. One might argue that with more patients and more healthcare provider included the system would have had a better chance to enfold its power. On the downside, the projects had inherent problems which could have maximised these deficiencies.

5. Conclusion

In response to the initial question "What went wrong in eMedCare?", there are three answers. The first point is that digital health is no solution but needs a shared and clear vision about the added value and an understanding of the processes required to achieve these goals. The second point is that each IT system must be evaluated for its usability in a given context. The final point is that the legal and technical framework provided by the national healthcare system must match the use cases envisioned. This applies to the German *Telematikinfrastruktur* on the part of the technology and the legal regulations of how physicians and nurses interact in primary care and how this is financially reimbursed.

Table 2: Comparison between selected NASSS criteria and the findings from the eMedCare project

	NASSS criteria	eMedCare
Technology:	*freestanding, not yet developed or fully interoperable;*	Tablet and portal software not integrated into IT system of the organisation; no relevant applications of the national *Telematikinfrastruktur* were available.
Organisation:	*Limited slack resources; Multiple organizations with partnership relationship; Some work needed to build shared vision, engage staff, enact new practices, and monitor impact*	IT system and processes increased the workload; there was no shared vision between nurses and physicians.
Value proposition:	*The value proposition of the technology was unclear, in terms of a viable business venture for its developer or in terms of a clear benefit for patients and an affordable real-world service model.*	The value proposition was unclear: The software provider originally pursued a different type of added value (mobile monitoring of patients) than the eMedCare consortium (communication). The value for the patient was never discussed.
Wider context:	*Complexity in external (financial, regulatory, legal, policy) issues—of which reimbursement seemed to be particularly key—stalled the mainstreaming and spread of the program.*	The interaction between nurses and physicians in primary care is regulated by the *Verordnung für Häusliche Krankenpflege* which does not include this general monitoring scenario for which the nurses did not get reimbursed.

Acknowledgement

We wish to thank Landkreis Osnabrück und Landkreis Emsland for supporting the evaluation study financially. We are also thankful for the contributions of the project participants. The overall project was financed by the State of Lower Saxony Germany and coordinated by the co-author MS.

Declarations

For both interview sessions a positive vote was obtained from the Ethics Commission of Hochschule Osnabrück (final VoteID: HSOS/2020/1/4).
The authors contributed to this study and this paper as follows:

- MP and LP: data gathering and analysis
- MP and UH: conceptualization and writing,
- LP, AB, and MS: review and editing.
- MS: project management
- UH, AB, and MS: supervision

References

[1]   Haggerty LJ, Reid RJ, Freeman GK, Starfield BH, Adair CE, McKendry R.: Continuity of care: a multidisciplinary review. BMJ. 2003;327:1219–1221.

[2]   Przysucha M, Vogel S, Hüsers J, Wache S, Sellemann B, Hübner U.: Requirements for Collaborative Decision Support Systems in Wound Care: No Information Continuity Without Management Continuity. Stud Health Technol Inform. 2018;253:133–137.

[3]   Sangaleti C, Schveitzer MC, Peduzzi M, Zoboli ELCP, and Soares CB. Experiences and shared meaning of teamwork and interprofessional collaboration among health care professionals in primary health care settings: a systematic review. JBI Database System Rev Implement Rep. 2017;15:2723–2788.

[4]   Garms-Homolová V.: Kooperation von Medizin und Pflege: Realisierbare Notwendigkeit oder unrealistischer Anspruch. In: Schaeffer D, Garms-Homolová V, editors: Medizin und Pflege. 1998; Ullstein Medical, Wiesbaden, p. 7–40.

[5]   Sachverständigenrat zur Begutachtung der Entwicklung im Gesundheitswesen. Gutachten 2007: Kooperation und Verantwortung. Voraussetzungen einer zielorientierten Gesundheitsversorgung, 2007.

[6]   Venkatesh V. Bala H.: Technology Acceptance Model 3 and a Research Agenda on Interventions. Decision Sciences. 2008;39:273–315.

[7]   Medifox, Medifox Wissensdatenbank, https://wissen.medifox.de/dashboard.action [cited 2022 May 11].

[8]   DM EDV, Das Konzept „ALLES AUS EINER HAND": So einfach wie nie!, 2015, https://silo.tips/download/das-konzept-alles-aus-einer-hand-so-einfach-wie-nie [cited 2022 May 11]

[9]   Mayring P.: Qualitative Inhaltsanalyse: Grundlagen und Techniken, 12th Edition. 2015. Beltz, Weinheim.

[10]   gematik GmbH: Alle Anwendungen: Die Zukunft des Gesundheitswesens ist digital, https://www.gematik.de/anwendungen/ [cited 2022 February 3].

[11]   Greenhalgh T, Wherton J, Papoutsi C, Lynch J, Hughes G, A'Court C et al.: Beyond Adoption: A New Framework for Theorizing and Evaluating Nonadoption, Abandonment, and Challenges to the Scale-Up, Spread, and Sustainability of Health and Care Technologies. J Med Internet Res. 2017;19:e367.

German Medical Data Sciences 2022 - Future Medicine
R. Röhrig et al. (Eds.)
© 2022 The authors and IOS Press.
This article is published online with Open Access by IOS Press and distributed under the terms
of the Creative Commons Attribution Non-Commercial License 4.0 (CC BY-NC 4.0).
doi:10.3233/SHTI220808

Usability of Electronic Health Records in Germany – An Overview of Satisfaction of University Hospital Physicians

Torben STÜER [a,1], and Christian JUHRA [a]

[a] *Office for eHealth, University Hospital Münster, Germany*

Abstract. Introduction: EHR are a part of daily task of physicians in Germany. This study surveyed the satisfaction of a small group of physicians in German university hospitals using EHR with focus on usability. Methods: The questioning was carried out by an online survey. Addressed were all physicians working at university hospitals in Germany. Results: The study showed that users are not satisfied with EHR (Grade 3.62). They pointed out some problems in general but reflected many advantages of those systems. Conclusion: EHR systems have to develop and adopt to users' tasks. They have to get faster and low error rates must be realized. Existing infrastructure must be improved and rolled out to users especially in times where digital healthcare services gain importance.

Keywords. electronic health record, EHR, usability, online survey, user experience, Survey, Germany, Finland, Denmark, digital healthcare services

1. Introduction

Electronic health records (EHR) support physicians at work every day. In Europe these systems are wide-spread and a shaping instrument of the daily clinic routine [1]. Simon [5] suspected a dissatisfaction among German physicians with those systems. The goal of this study was to gather an overview about satisfaction of physicians with direct patient contact in Germany. We wanted to get an up-to-date picture specifically focused on usability. In current literature there is no such data for physicians in Germany but in Finland [2] and Denmark [17]. In this study we adapted the study from Finland and carried out an online survey addressed to all physicians at university hospitals in Germany. Furthermore, the goal was to compare the findings of our study to the results from Denmark [17] and Finland [2] as already discussed in 2017 [6].

2. Background

An important factor in user satisfaction with a software system is user experience, more specifically usability. The relevance of usability of software usability was taken into consideration early. Both generally [7] and in more specific aspects [8,9,10]. It is also a factor to user acceptance [11,12]. Usability is defined in ISO 9241-11:2018 [13] as:

---
[1] Corresponding Author: Torben Stüer, Office for eHealth, University Hospital Münster, Albert-Schweitzer-Campus 1, 48149 Münster, Germany; Email: torbenstueer@uni-muenster.de.

„the extent to which a system, product or service can be used by specified users to achieve specified goals with effectiveness, efficiency and satisfaction in a specified context of use". To review the usability of a piece of software there are three guiding criteria [2]:

- effectiveness
- efficiency
- satisfaction

in a specified context of use.

In 2010 a study was designed in Finland with the aim of investigating and measuring the usability and user experiences of EHRs [2] and gather information on users' experiences with these systems focused on usability. The guiding criteria were transformed into three special factors which became the basis of the questions posed in the study:

1. Compatibility between physician task and the EHR system (productivity).
2. Information exchange, communication and collaboration (between different user groups e.g. physicians, nurses and patients).
3. Interoperability (between different systems and external software) and reliability.

The study addressed all physicians in all sectors of the healthcare system in Finland and showed a dissatisfaction among participants interacting with EHRs. Repeat studies were conducted in 2014 and 2017. These showed that the overall satisfaction of participants has not improved over the years. Users in hospitals and healthcare centers do not feel EHRs support them in their work. In contrast, satisfaction with usability in hospitals has improved. In 2017 it was suggested that the lack of progress is a result of the implementation of National Health Information Services [6]. In Denmark, another country leading in healthcare digitization, Christian Nøhr carried out a similar survey in 2018. He addressed all medical professionals (nurses, medical secretaries, physicians and radiographers). The results showed that satisfaction differs depending on region, used system and the respondents' career group [17]. Prior to the study discussed in this paper, no such study of EHR usability has been conducted in Germany.

3. Material and methods

This survey is based on the study by Viitanen [2] in 2010. The original study was designed as an online survey. This type of data collection ensured a high degree of availability to participants, easy access from any computer, and data that was easy and quick to evaluate and compare. Furthermore, it is also considered a cost-effective method [14]. For the study's German adaption, we chose the same method and tried to reach a large number of participants. In Germany there is no central register of email addresses belonging to physicians and to further complicate the matter not every physician (392,492 at the end of 2018 [15]) has an email address. A paper-based or interview-based study was not a reasonable alternative as these methods are both very time consuming and expensive. First, we tried unsuccessfully to contact all physicians in Germany via the German medical association. We then reduced our peer group and tried to reach all physicians working at a university hospital in Germany via the corresponding central departments for information technology. There was never any direct contact between us and any potential respondents, and the number of physicians working at university hospitals is not information available to public, hence why we are not able to declare a response rate. We created an email to contact potential participants and explained what the study is about and what the goal of our research is. An email address was made available, but not used by participants, for questions. Time required to complete the whole survey was approximated to be 15 minutes. It could be stopped and restarted at any point. We asked the corresponding head of information technology to forward the email to the corresponding emailing list for all physicians. We also asked to remind users to answer one week before the study ended. Just as the original study from Finland, the survey starts with a question as to whether or not the participant works in direct patient contact followed by 11 questions about their general background and 5 about EHR experience. Next, 37 questions on hospital information systems, two questions concerning the pros and cons of working with EHRs., followed by a space for feedback at the end. Most of these were single-choice questions on a five-point Likert scale ("Agree fully to" to "Do not agree at all"). A question about the overall rating was asked using common German school grades (1 - 6). This structure and the possibility to give feedback at the end of the survey enabled the participants to provide both negative and positive response. Just as in the surveys in Finland and Denmark, 8 questions were aimed specifically at the usability of the EHR:

1. The arrangement of fields and functions on the computer screen is logical
2. Terminology on the screen is clear and understandable
3. Entering patient data is easy and quick
4. Routine tasks can be performed in a straight forward manner without the need for extra steps
5. It is easy to obtain the patient information that I need
6. The system responds quickly to inputs
7. Faulty system function has caused or has nearly caused a serious adverse event for the patient
8. Information systems help in preventing errors and mistakes associated with medications

For easier access for German users, we translated the original study from Finland [2] into German and adapted the study to German conditions.

4. Implementation

We used LimeSurvey 3.14.5 [18] for standardized implementation and visualization for participants. The Website was hosted by the University Hospital Münster, Institute of Medical Informatics. In May 2018 we started piloting at University Hospital Münster. Respondents did not report encountering issues, so no changes needed to be made in implementation. Other university hospitals followed in December 2018 and January 2019. SPSS 25.0 [16] was used for statistical analysis. A descriptive analysis of data was conducted and only physicians with direct patient contact which completed the whole study were included in the evaluation. The selection was made by controlling the answer to the first question in the survey.

5. Results

Only 139 participants visited the landing page of the survey. 72 (52%) stopped after the first question about patient contact. 69 (48%) started the survey, work in direct contact with patients and filled out the survey completely. Only they were included into the evaluation. The demographic distribution shows a young respondent group (Mean 42 years) (see figure 1).

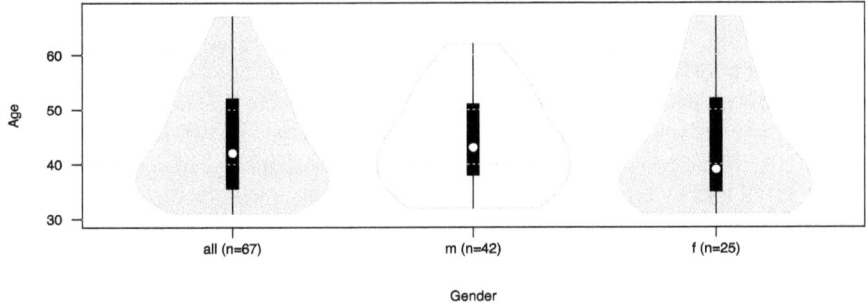

Figure 1. Demography of participants

We received from three different university hospitals working with either Cerner Medico (n=30, 45%) or Dedalus Orbis (n=37, 55%). 29 of 69 (42%) had no specialist title at the time of this survey. The most represented field of specialization was anesthesia and intensive care (n= 21, 30%), followed by internal medicine (n=5, 7%) and pediatrics (n=5, 7%). 30 % (n=20) worked in the operating room or in an outpatient department, and 9% (n=6) in an intensive care unit. 67 (100%) participants rated the current EHR system used in their hospital a mean 3.62 (1 = excellent, 6 = fail) (Range 6, min 1, max 6, Std. Dev. 1.23).

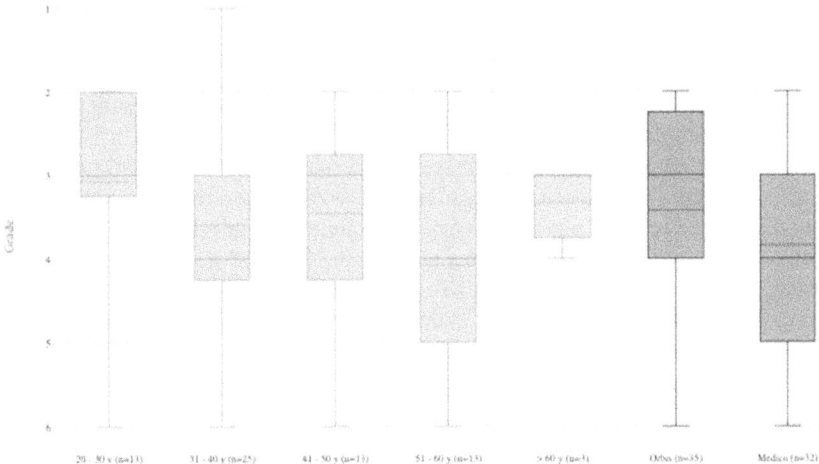

Figure 2. Overview of overall grade by grade and used EHR

A deviation of the participants final grade showed up in the age group of 20 - 30 years and a slight deviation in the overall score between the different EHR systems. It is interesting that 64 of 67 (95%) respondents classified themselves as being averagely experienced at using EHR systems and 51 of 67 (76%) have been using the current EHR system for more than 3 years. The longer participants use a system the lower they tend to grade it. The mean decreased from 2,3 (<1/2 year, n=3) to 3.75 (>6 years, n=37). 64% (n=43) have experience with two or more EHR systems and are able comparison. Most participants (n=46, 69%) agreed that an EHR is helpful in their everyday work. They frequently praised the availability of patient information regardless of physician´s location (n=26, 39%), management of work (n=15, 22%9 and digital dictation (n=14, 21%).

The primary goal of this study was to get an overview of user satisfaction with a focus on usability. Figure 3 shows no clear answer to this question because participants' answers differ a lot. However, 67% (n=45) stated that routine tasks cannot be performed in straightforward manner. 55% (n=37) state that faulty system functions (nearly) caused serious adverse effects to patients and 55% (n=37) not content with the input-response of their EHR. These two points are a sign of poor technical quality. As a benefit of EHRs 49% (n=33) of users were prevented from making mistakes with medication.

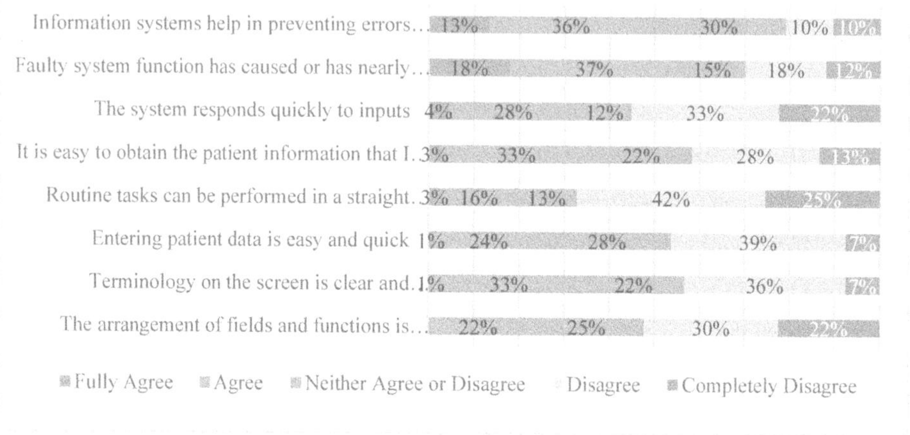

Information systems help in preventing errors… 13% | 36% | 30% | 10% | 10%

Faulty system function has caused or has nearly… 18% | 37% | 15% | 18% | 12%

The system responds quickly to inputs 4% | 28% | 12% | 33% | 22%

It is easy to obtain the patient information that I… 3% | 33% | 22% | 28% | 13%

Routine tasks can be performed in a straight… 3% | 16% | 13% | 42% | 25%

Entering patient data is easy and quick 1% | 24% | 28% | 39% | 7%

Terminology on the screen is clear and… 1% | 33% | 22% | 36% | 7%

The arrangement of fields and functions is… 22% | 25% | 30% | 22%

■ Fully Agree   ■ Agree   ■ Neither Agree or Disagree   Disagree   ■ Completely Disagree

Figure 3. Overview Usability aimed questions

Communication and data exchange between different hospitals or with the outpatient sector is as an important factor in the future. Respondents stated that it is still primary done via email (93%, n=62) or fax (64%, n=43). Teleradiological networks (21%, n=14)) and upload portals (27%, n=18) are used much less often for exchanging data. While the ability to cooperate with physicians from different hospitals was rated poorly (58%, n=39), cooperation between physicians at the same hospital was rated much better and 84% (n=56) of the participants are satisfied. Overall, the open feedback rate was high at 34% (n=23). Consensus among participants´ comments was that their EHR seemed slow (55%, n=37) and the user interface was unintuitive. Only 46% (n=31) of users rated their EHR system as stable.

6. Discussion and Conclusion

In this study we aimed to get an overview of EHRs satisfaction among physicians in Germany who have direct patient contact. We failed to meet this goal because we had to shrink the target-group to physicians working at a university hospital and the number of participants was very low. It is therefore not possible to make any general claims about EHR-satisfaction based on the results. Due to the number of physicians working at university hospitals being an unknown number, we are not able to declare a response rate. We do however suspect it is low. This limits the reliability of this study. We encountered many issues trying to get in contact with physicians. In Germany there is no database of email address for every physician accessible. For instance, there is no central register with physicians' email addresses in Germany. Even the chosen method of communication via emailing lists and the aid of the head of information technology was difficult. We do not know if every physician in the corresponding hospital was reached. Email is not optimal to contact participants to answer a survey [19] but we choose it anyway because the realization of a paper-based study or invitation would have been much more expensive and would likely have failed. Nevertheless, we were able to get an overview of opinions within out small group of respondents. In this group EHR systems are perceived as helpful in their everyday clinical routine. However, users are not satisfied with these systems in general (Grade 3.62). The grade given differs depending on system used and usage time. EHR-satisfaction was expected to differ depending on what EHR-systems respondents use. We did not expect a correlation between dissatisfaction with an EHR and usage time. We expected that users would adapt to and accept the problems of that EHR-system over time. Instead, they grow increasingly dissatisfied the longer they interact with it. Special interest was paid to the age group of 21-30 years (grade 3.07). We purpose that this group, also known as digital natives, have had much more access to and experience with technology and therefore solve problems in a more intuitive way. The second important aspect of this study was the focus on usability. Users have voiced their dissatisfaction with the perceived poor technical quality of EHR systems. Developers are the ones tasked with solving this and should aim to make EHR systems more stable and less error-prone. Likewise, users criticized how sluggish EHR-systems felt to use. Users and patients rely on EHR-systems and despite the fact no generalized evaluation of the ease of use could be conducted we found that users do not feel well supported in general by EHR-systems in their clinical routine. In order to tackle these issues, there needs to be clear and constructive communication between developers and users. The usability of software always depends on whether it fits the context of use. Accurate mapping of everyday work and routines to a system-interface requires a lot of communication between software developers and physicians. This process begins with setting up and do not end with maintaining an EHR. Finally, our goal was to compare our data to the results from Finland and Denmark. As mentioned by Viitanen et al [6] in 2018. The structure of the survey enabled a caparison of the satisfaction with the usability of EHR systems in Finland, Germany and Denmark. However, a direct comparison was not possible because the studies addressed different participants and the sample size in Germany was very small and could not be generalized. Furthermore, usability is not numerical so it cannot be compared easily. We tried to highlight some of the important differences. Finland's participants ascribe their EHR a good ease of use. Arrangement of fields seems to be much better in Finland as the support for routine tasks. Moreover, in Finland and Denmark system-errors and less speed are not commonly cited problems. German users, in contrast, are very happy with the EHRs ability to prevent medication-related errors and feel EHRs are very useful in that context. This study was designed and carried out in 2018/2019, and published in 2022. This means that the results may not necessarily reflect the current state of things. Nevertheless, it gives an overview of satisfaction among physicians with focus on usability. Some points have improved in the meantime but many issues remain [20]. For example, during the Covid 19 pandemic sick leave by telephone was possible. It was not the goal of this study to solve the problems of EHR systems. However, if you look to Denmark or Finland some points are rated better in those countries than in Germany. It may be useful to look to them in order to find solutions for our EHR-related problems by examining how those functions were implemented differently over there.

7. Outlook

This study provided an insight into the experiences of survey respondents with their current EHR system in German university hospitals. EHRs are an important part of everyday clinical routine with many pros and cons. Digitalization in healthcare and the importance of EHR will increase. To further the development of EHR existing infrastructure has to be implemented. A good infrastructure has been laid by the Gematik group. This group was founded in 2005 and deploys a telematic infrastructure e.g. e-prescription, data exchange (ISIK, KIM (i.e. communication in medicine) or ePA. This basic infrastructure has only been slowly adopted by the developers of EHRs and has not become widespread among medical professionals or patients. After the implementation many of these problems will be solved but some might also give rise to new problems. New devices (e.g. tablets) will expand the range of applications for EHR systems. For better user acceptance of "classic" EHR and new mobile solutions it is crucial to improve the usability. Developers have to decrease errors and to raise speed of EHRs. In private sector users see that the software is high responsive, works with low error rate and good usability. Users want this at work and in especially in EHR systems. To solve this problem the communication between the users and the developers of the software seems to be particularly important and an important part of the solution. Since this study is the first survey of its kind in Germany, it would be useful to have a follow-up study with a larger sample-size. Similar to the studies in Finland, it would be interesting to see user-satisfaction as well as new problems or worsening of the situation.

Author´s contribution

TS: conception and implementation of study, Adaptation of study design, data collection and interpretation, writing of manuscript;
CJ: conception and implementation of study, quality control reworking of the manuscript;
All authors have approved the manuscript as submitted and assume responsibility for the scientific integrity of the work.

Conflicts of interest

All authors declare that they have no conflicts of interest.

Acknowledgement

We would like to thank Johanna Viitanen (Department of Computer Science, Espoo, Aalto University, Finland) for the idea and conception [2,4,6] and to make available data. In this context we would like to thank Christian Nøhr (Institut for Planlægning, Aalborg, Aalborg University, Denmark) for data from Denmark (not yet published but presented on UTCH 2019). For hosting the study we would like to thank the Institute of Medical Informatics, University of Münster.

References

[1] C. Codagnone and F. Lupiañez-Villanueva, Benchmarking deployment of eHealth among general practitioners (2013): Final report, Publications Office European Commission, Luxembourg, 2013.

[2] J. Viitanen, H. Hyppönen, T. Lääveri, J. Vänskä, J. Reponen, and I. Winblad, National questionnaire study on clinical ICT systems proofs: Physicians suffer from poor usability, International Journal of Medical Informatics. 80 (2011) 708–725. doi:10.1016/j.ijmedinf.2011.06.010

[3] T. Vehko, S. Ruotsalainen, H. Hyppönen, E-health and e-welfare of Finland, Checkpoint 2018, National Institute for Health and Welfare (THL). Helsinki, Finland (2019). ISBN 978-952-343-325-0 (printed); ISBN 978-952-343-326-7 (pdf).

[4] J. Kaipio, T. Lääveri, H. Hyppönen, S. Vainiomäki, J. Reponen, A. Kushniruk, E. Borycki, and J. Vänskä, Usability problems do not heal by themselves: National survey on physicians' experiences with EHRs in Finland, International Journal of Medical Informatics. 97 (2017) 266–281. doi:10.1016/j.ijmedinf.2016.10.010.

[5] A. Simon, Wie zufrieden sind Anwender mit der IT-Unterstützung im Krankenhaus? Pilotstudie zur empirischen Erhebung und Validierung der allgemeinen Zufriedenheit von IT-Anwendern im Krankenhaus, GMS Medizinische Informatik. (2017) Biometrie und Epidemiologie; 13(1). doi:10.3205/MIBE000171.

[6] J. Kaipio, H. Hyppönen, andT. Lääveri, Physicians' Experiences on EHR Usability: A Time Series from 2010, 2014 and 2017. in Improving Usability, Safety and Patient Outcomes with Health Information Technology. Studies in Health Technology and Informatics, vol. 257 (2019), https://doi.org/10.3233/978-1-61499-951-5-194

[7] J. Nielsen, Usability engineering, 3rd Edition, Kaufmann, Amsterdam, Heidelberg, 2010

[8] J. Belden, R. Grayson, J. Barnes, Defining and testing EMR usability: principles and proposed methods of EMR usability evaluation and rating, Healthcare Information and Management Systems Society, Chicago, USA, 2009.

[9] R. Schumacher, J. Webb and J. Johnson, How to Select an Electronic Health Record System that Healthcare Professionals can Use, User Centric, Oakbrook Terrace, USA, 2009.

[10] D. Svanaes, A. Das, and O.A. Alsos, The contextual nature of usability and its relevance to medical informatics. Stud Health Technol Inform 136 (2008), 541–546.

[11] H.L. Bleich, and W.V. Slack, Reflections on electronic medical records: When doctors will use them and when they will not, International Journal of Medical Informatics. 79 (2010) 1–4. doi:10.1016/j.ijmedinf.2009.10.002.

[12] M. Zahabi, D.B. Kaber, and M. Swangnetr, Usability and Safety in Electronic Medical Records Interface Design, Hum Factors. 57 (2015) 805–834. doi:10.1177/0018720815576827.

[13] International Organization for Standardization, ISO 9241-11:2018: Ergonomics of human-system interaction — Part 11: Usability: Definitions and concepts, Geneva, Switzerland. https://www.iso.org/obp/ui/#iso:std:iso:9241:-11:ed-2:v1:en (accessed May 1, 2022).

[14] J. Kirakowski, Questionnaires in usability engineering - A List of Frequently Asked Questions, (2019 http://edutechwiki.unige.ch/en/Usability_and_user_experience_surveys (accessed May 1, 2022).

[15] Bundesärztekammer Deutschland, Ärztestatistik zum 31. Dezember 2018, Berlin, Germany. https://www.bundesaerztekammer.de/ueber-uns/aerztestatistik/aerztestatistik-2018/ (accessed May 1, 2022).

[16] IBM Corp (2017) IBM SPSS Statistics, IBM Corp, Armonk, NY.

[17] C. Juhra, J. Viitanen, C. Nøhr, Usability of Hospital Information Systems - Challenges for the Future (2019), ITCH 2019 (Victoria(BC)), Canada.

[18] Limesurvey GmbH, LimeSurvey: An Open Source survey tool, LimeSurvey GmbH, Hamburg, Germany. http://www.limesurvey.org (accessed May 1, 2022).

[19] J. Sitzia, and N. Wood, Response rate in patient satisfaction research: an analysis of 210 published studies, International Journal for Quality in Health Care. 10 (1998) 311–317. doi:10.1093/intqhc/10.4.311.

[20] U. Hübner, M. Esdar, J Hüsers, JD. Liebe, L. Naumann, J. Thye, JP. Weiß. IT-Report Gesundheitswesen, Schwerpunkt - Wie reif ist die Gesundheits-IT aus Anwenderperspektive?, Forschungsgruppe Informatik im Gesundheitswesen (IGW), Schriftenreihe der Hochschule Osnabrück, Germany (2020), ISBN 978-3-9817805-2-9, 331

German Medical Data Sciences 2022 - Future Medicine
R. Röhrig et al. (Eds.)
© 2022 The authors and IOS Press.
doi:10.3233/SHTI220809

Assessment of the Consistency of Categorical Features Within the DZHK Biobanking Basic Set

Khalid YUSUF [a*], Kais TAHAR[a*], Ulrich SAX[a,b], Wolfgang HOFFMANN[c,d], and
Dagmar KREFTING[a,b,c,1]

[a]Department of Medical Informatics, University Medical Center Göttingen,
Göttingen,Germany
[b]Campus Institute Data Science (CIDAS), Georg August-University, Göttingen,
Germany
[c]DZHK (German Centre for Cardiovascular Research)
[d]Institute for Community Medicine, Department Epidemiology of Health Care and
Community Health, University Medicine Greifswald, Germany

Abstract
Data quality in health research encompasses a broad range of aspects and indicators.
While some indicators are generic and can be calculated without domain knowledge,
others require information about a specific data element. Even more complex are
indicators addressing contradictions, that stem from implausible combinations of
multiple data elements. In this paper, we investigate how contradictions within
interdependent categorical data can be identified and if they give additional
information about possible quality issues, their cause, and mitigation options. The
19 data elements that represent four biosample types including their pre-analytic
states within the DZHK Biobanking basic set are exported to the CDISC Operational
Data Model (ODM), transformed and loaded into a tranSMART instance. Through
the implementation of a data quality assessment workflow as a SmartR plug-in,
statistical information about the domain-specific consistency of interdependent
values are retrieved, assessed, and visualized. Data quality indicators have been
selected for the assessment according to common recommendations found in the
literature. Different contradictions could be discovered in the dataset including
mismatch of interdependent values in the pre-analytic states of blood and urine
samples, as well as primary and aliquoted samples. The overall assessment rating
shows that 99.61% of the interdependent values are free of contradictions. However,
measures within the EDC design to avoid contradictions may result in overestimated
missing rates in automatic, item-based quality assessment checks. Through
consistency checks on interdependent categorical features, we demonstrated that
consistency flaws can be found in the categorical data of biobanking metadata and
that they can help to detect issues in the data entry process. Our approach
underscores the importance of domain knowledge in the definition of the
consistency rules but also knowledge about the EDC implementation of such
consistency rules to consider the impact on item-based quality indicators.

Keywords. Data quality, Biological specimen bank, metadata

---

* The first two authors should be regarded as joint first authors.

1 University Medical Center Göttingen, Germany; E-mail: dagmar.krefting@med.uni-goettingen.de.

1. Introduction

Data quality in health research encompasses a broad range of aspects and indicators [1-3]. According to [1], the DIN (German Institute for Standardization) EN ISO 14050 2010, defines the term data quality as the "properties of data with regard to their suitability for fulfilling specified requirements". Thus, quality indicators are quantifiable measures to describe data quality for a specific purpose. Some indicators are generic and can be calculated without domain knowledge, e.g. the completeness of a mandatory data element within a data set. Others require information about a specific data element, for example, to define limits for acceptable values. Even more complex are indicators addressing contradictions, that stem from implausible combinations of multiple data elements. A typical example is the rule, that the diastolic blood pressure must not be higher than the systolic blood pressure when measured simultaneously.

A key asset of the DZHK is the DZHK Heart Bank that provides liquid biomaterial samples and image data with comprehensive clinical data for research projects from all studies directly funded[2]. A common data set encompassing clinical data and the metadata describing the available bio-samples and images has been defined that allows interested researchers to access this information throughout the Heart Bank. The definition of the data elements including the Biobanking basic set (BBS) can be found in the publicly available data catalogue[3]. Biomaterial can be considered as a specifically valuable asset due to its high processing and maintenance costs as well as their finite nature - other than digital data, that can be copied without loss. Therefore, accuracy of associated data is of high importance, in particular in scientific cohort studies and registries [1]. To encourage consistency in the collection of high-quality data associated with biomaterial, Kiehntopf and Böer recommend data reconciliation techniques to be introduced in the biobank's information system [4, p. 64]. Previous studies have shown instances of data anomalies in biomaterial banks [5,6]. Also, the pre-analytic states of blood samples have been observed as one of the leading sources of errors in clinical laboratories [7,8]. As the DZHK BBS encompasses information about the different states of the samples, we implemented a data quality workflow to assess potential contradictions regarding the biosample processing states.

2. Material and Methods

2.1. Data

The Translational Registry for Cardiomyopathies (TORCH) has been one of the first registries conducted within the DZHK. It encompasses comprehensive data of 2300 patients with non-ischemic cardiomyopathies in order to analyze the parthenogenesis and therapeutic interventions for cardiomyopathy patients [9]. The data is recorded using the Electronic Data Capture (EDC) System secuTrial, including the BBS for this registry. Since most variables in biomaterial data are categorical, our case study investigates the categorical data elements within the BBS that capture information about EDTA (ethylenediaminetetraacetic acid) plasma, citrate plasma, serum, and urine. For each of

---

2 https://dzhk.de/en/dzhk-heart-bank/daten-und-bioproben/ressource-mit-fluessigproben-und-bilddaten/
3 https://dzhk.de/en/research/data-and-sample-collections/data-catalogue/biobanking-basic-set/

these sample types, three data elements refer to them: The number of primary receptables filled, that may range from 0 to 2, where 2 is only allowed in EDTA and Citrate plasma if the biomaterial kit is from specific manufacturer. The content of the primary receptables is then distributed to aliquots of 300 ul. For each sample type, a desired number of aliquots is defined. The second and the third data elements refer to the number of the filled aliquots: One element represents the fact, that all desired aliquots are filled, while the other element represents the quantity of aliquots filled if the desired number of aliquots is not reached. We also investigate the data elements that capture the pre-analytic properties of blood and urine samples. For blood, the four possible states are *normal, lipeamic, icteric* and *haemolytic*. They are determined by the color of the blood plasma. For urine, three different states are addressed: *normal, cloudy* and *bloody*, and are also determined by visual inspection. A total of 19 categorical elements are thus considered.

2.2. Selection of Data Quality Indicators

Two factors have been considered in the selection of data quality indicators for the assessment of consistency as follows: (1) The quality indicators are described consistently in current literature and (2) they are suitable for interdependent data elements. Among the prominent data quality metrics that feature mostly in literature are those identified in the data quality assessment guidelines by the TMF (Technology and Method Platform for Networked Medical Research) team [1] and the harmonized framework by Kahn et al. [2]. Schmidt et al. [3] also formulated a harmonized framework at the intersection of [1] and [2]. These resources were considered in the determination of suitable indicators for the assessment of the consistency of interdependent categorical features. Two data quality indicators are considered within the taxonomy of Schmidt et al: (1) logical contradictions, and (2) empirical contradictions. The primary reporting metrics of the indicators are thus the number of data fields N and the rate of inconsistent data %. This is also in accordance with the recommendation by Nonnemacher et al. [1]. An alternative definition of these quality indicators has been proposed by Kahn et al.: Atemporal plausibility through (a) common and (b) domain knowledge. While the latter would better reflect the atemporal character of the assessment, the former better reflects the aspect of a multi-item based quality indicator. Our decision is based on the consideration that the present work focuses on categorical variables thus excluding time-related aspects, and exclusively addresses multi-item contradictions.

2.3. Data Quality Assessment implementation in tranSMART

The data has been exported in secutrial's built-in ODM format and transformed to be loaded into the tranSMART (v16.2) analysis platform through its standard *batch_importer* method. The data quality assessment workflow is developed as a SmartR plug-in. SmartR plug-ins allow for the application of arbitrary operations on data stored in tranSMART [10]. Through the logical rules implemented in the R-Script components of the plug-in, interdependent data elements are tested against predefined logic. An inference is drawn by combining results from the data analysis with the common knowledge from the study design and domain knowledge offered by the experts. The statistical information derived from the R-Script analysis is then written as JSON object and parsed to the built-in D3-js component for visualization.

3. Results

3.1. Consistency between primary receptables and sample aliquots

As explained in section 2.1, figure 1 describes the flow of interdependent fields within the three data elements of each sample type: The number of primary receptables, the information if the desired number of aliquots are available, and - if the latter is not the case, the number of aliquots filled. In the paper-based Biomaterial Collection Form Basis Set, the number of primary receptables can be set to 0, 1 and additionally for plasma 2. For the aliquot number, there is a tickbox that allows to mark that all aliquots area filled. The number of desired aliquots is given besides the tickbox. Besides the tickbox, a field is given, with a header "Quantity". In the electronic form, in addition to the possible categorical values described above, further options not known (unbekannt) and not ascertained (nicht erhoben) are implemented for all items. The form has been implemented in a way, that the number of aliquots (Aliquot count) is only visible if the checkbox is set to no. Missing values are indicated by NA. The combinations of contradictory values are given in Table 1.

Nr. of primary receptables   All aliquots filled   Aliquot count

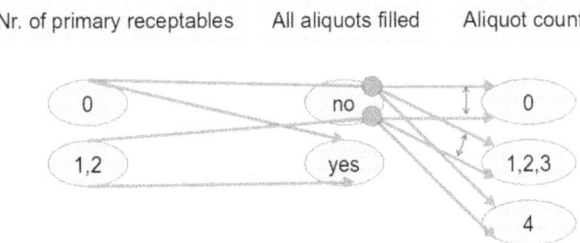

Figure 1: Flow of interdependent fields in the case report form (CRF). Impossible combinations due to implemented rules are not shown. Green arrows indicate plausible combinations, red arrows implausible combinations of item values. Violet arrow indicates combinations where plausibility can only be determined if the Nr. of primary receptables is considered, thus indicating a multidimensional consistency.

Table 1: Contradictory values in sample type quantities.

Rule	Nr. of Primary Receptables	All aliquots filled	Aliquot count
C1	0	yes	NA
C2	0	no	>0
C3	>0	yes	< desired aliquots
C4	>0	no	desired aliquots

Figure 2 shows the visualization of the data quality assessment for citrate plasma within tranSMART. For citrate, the maximum number of primary receptables is 2, and the number of desired aliquots is 4. For the visualization of the three dimensions a tile-based plot has been chosen. The color of the tile indicates the consistency, the number within the tile indicates the number of datasets where this value combination is found. Contradictions C1 and C2 are found in the left column of the tile matrix (*Primary receptables = 0*), C4 is found in the 2nd and 3rd column (*Primary receptables = 1,2*) within the 2nd row (*aliquot_nein*), although in very few cases. We would like to note that by EDC design, C3 is already inhibited, because the number of aliquots cannot be entered if the status that all aliquots are filled is set to *yes*. This implies that in the majority of cases, the value for the Aliquot count is NA. Naive counting of NA values in individual data elements for completeness would result here in a high number of missing values. Another aspect is the handling of implausible combinations that are caused by missing values. In the last column (Primary receptables = NA) some entries for a full as well as an incomplete aliquot set can be observed. However, we have decided to count such implausibilities not as contradiction, as it would consider a missing value in the same way as an entered value.

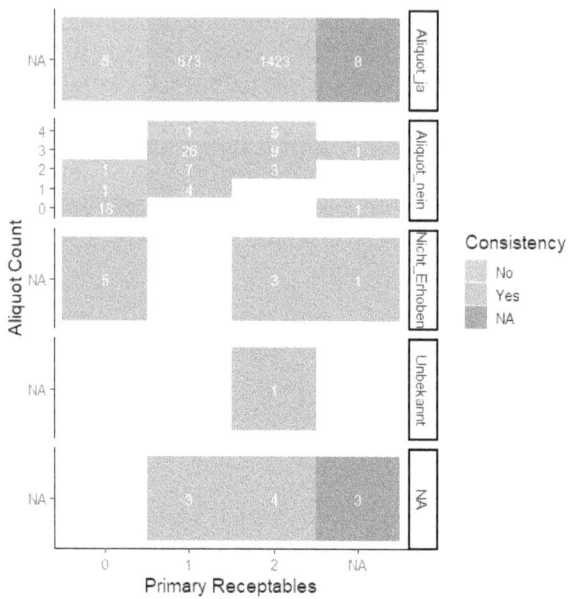

Figure 2: Visualization of the quality indicator consistency for citrate samples. Tiles represent the different states of the item value combinations; the color indicates the result of the consistency evaluation and the number gives the number found within the respective tile. (NA = missing).

3.2. Consistency of the pre-analytic sample states

The pre-analytic states of blood and urine both depend on the visual inspection of the respective liquid sample. The following combinations are inconsistent: All states are set to *no*, normal state and at least one other state are set to *yes*. According to domain expert, combinations of the states *lipemic, icteric and hemolytic* are consistent for blood samples and combinations of *cloudy* and *bloody* are consistent for urine samples.

The paper-based form has three tick-boxes for each property: *yes, no,* and *not ascertained*. Again, missing values are represented by NA in the electronic form. Furthermore, the states other than normal are only shown if normal is not set to yes, impeding the inconsistency that normal state and at least one other state are set to *yes*. Figure 3 shows the visualization for the blood sample properties. Here, combinations of four items are visualized. Only item values are shown that appear at least once in the respective combination. For example, the value *not ascertained (nicht erhoben)* is only found in combinations where all four properties are not ascertained and in one case, where hemolytic state is set to yes and all others to not ascertained. Due to the implemented consistency rule within the electronic form, all other states are set to NA if state normal is set to yes. Again, we find the possible inconsistency where all states are set to *no* but again in very few cases. Again, for the vast majority of cases, the possibility to create inconsistent combinations of values has been prevented by EDC design: Values for diverging blood properties cannot be set if the property *normal* has been set to *yes*. As the paper-based form explicitly asks for individual assessment of each of the properties including the option to set *not ascertained* for each property, without knowledge of the EDC rules, the NA values for the diverging properties might be interpreted as missing in completeness assessments. Domain experts evaluated it as implausible that the blood-state is not ascertained at all, but we did not consider it here as contradictory, as *not ascertained* is a valid value.

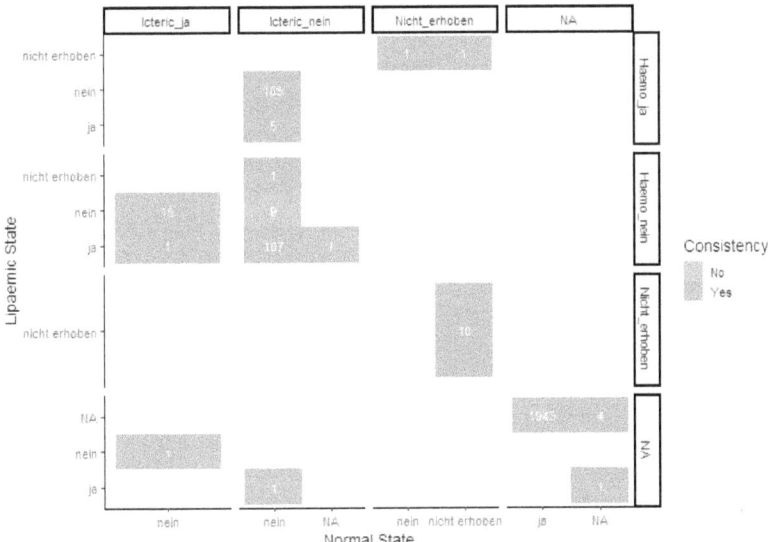

Figure 3: Visualization of the consistency of pre-analytic states of blood samples. Tiles represent the combination of the four different variables, indicated at the four axes. (haemo:hemolytic state, ja: yes, nein:no, nicht erhoben: not ascertained, NA: missing)

3.3. Overall Quality Assessment Report

The quality of the TORCH categorical dataset is assessed using the atemporal consistency metric for all mentioned variables. The overall assessment rating, given in Table 2, shows that 99.61% of the interdependent fields are free of contradictions. The consistency rates for different classes of interdependent categorical features are all in the same order of magnitude and show very few consistency flaws. We would like to mention that here the number of affected fields, i.e. the individual data item values are given rather than the number of inconsistent value combinations. The number of actual datasets that contain inconsistencies and may therefore not be used is obtained by the division of the number of variables involved (4 for blood-states, 3 for others).

Table 2: Data Quality Assessment Report. (AC = Atemporal Consistency)

Feature	ConsistencyCheck			
	Passed-Fields	Failed-Fields	Plausible-Rate (%)	
EDTA	6600	18	99.73	
Serum	6612	6	99.91	
Citrat	6579	39	99.41	Logical contradictions
Urine	6567	51	99.23	
Urine-states	6603	15	99.77	
Blood-states	8788	36	99.59	Empirical contradictions
Summary	41749	165	99.61	

4. Discussion

The present work considers multi-directional consistency checks to detect inconsistencies within interdependent data elements in a biomaterial variable set. This approach helps to assess the consistency of interdependent values in three-way relationships (as seen in section 3.1) and four-way relationships (as demonstrated in section 3.2). With this approach we go beyond the item-based consistency checks for example executed in the works of Spengler et al. [11] and Blacketer et al. [12] and that are common in EDC design. Schmidt et al. [3] considered consistency checks involving two data values of the same measurement unit using their *con_contradictions* module in *DataquieR* package, but this is still not sufficient to check for multi-directional consistency issues across multiple interdependent elements as obtained in this study. While the quality indicators defined in this work fit well into the proposed taxonomy by Schmidt et al. [3], in future work, we would explore how the *con_contradictions* module can be adapted to fit specific consistency requirements like we have in our use case. The main contribution of our work is the assessment of multi-item contradictions in a dataset. In the investigated TORCH study, EDC design already prevents main multi-item contradictions by hiding parts of the form if a specific condition is set. However, in the current implementation *NAs* resulting from a conditional rule and *NAs* resulting from missing information can only be distinguished by knowledge of the specific rules. For automatic assessment of item-based quality indicators such as completeness it might be helpful to have a specific value that indicates that the item could not be entered in this case due to EDC rules, e.g. *not shown*. Also, unrestricted fields as observed in the entry of the count of aliquots will result in the entry of arbitrary values that can contradict other predefined dependent values in other elements.

Consistency checks on contradictions have shown to require domain and process knowledge but also knowledge about the EDC implementation. The implemented checks are specific to DZHK biomaterial data. Hence, more collaboration with domain experts is needed to specify convenient rules for other use cases. As we found very few remaining contradictions in the data set, a concrete benefit of the effort for the improvement of the quality of the TORCH data set might be disputable. But we would like to emphasize, that the strength of the DZHK Heart bank lies in the harmonization of processes and data sets. Therefore, the implemented quality indicators are applicable to all DZHK-funded studies.

5. Conclusion

We demonstrate methods and tools for interactive data quality reviews. These are of utmost importance for improving single data sets and especially integrated data sets. Through consistency assessment on interdependent categorical items, data quality flaws could be identified in the DZHK-BBS. Our results underscore the importance of domain knowledge in both the clinical aspects but also in the aspects of information system design for data quality assessment.

Declarations

Ethical approval and consent: Use of the TORCH dataset was approved by DZHK and TORCH.

Conflict of Interest: The authors declare, that there is no conflict of interest.

Author Contributions: This paper is based on the master thesis of KY (Master's Graduate), he conceived the study together with KT, US and DK (Supervisors). KY handled the software implementation and data analysis. KT performed the use case selection and requirement analysis as well as the software design and the supervision of practical implementation. WH contributed expertise in domain related questions. KY, KT and DK formulated the manuscript with contributions from all authors.

Acknowledgement: The work is supported by the German Centre for Cardiovascular research (DZHK). We equally recognize the support of Ms. Otte, the Chief Laboratory Technician at the UMG.

Availability of data and materials: The used data is available within the DZHK Heart bank[4] available for researchers through the common DZHK Use & Access process. The source-code of the plug-in implementation is publicly available in the Gitlab repository of the project[5].

References

[1]   M. Nonnemacher, D. Nasseh, J. Stausberg, and U. Bauer, *Datenqualität in der medizinischen Forschung: Leitlinie zum adaptiven Management von Datenqualität in Kohortenstudien und Registern*, 2., Aktualisierte und erw. Aufl. Berlin: Med. Wiss. Verl.- Ges, 2014.

[2]   M. G. Kahn *et al.*, "A Harmonized Data Quality Assessment Terminology and Framework for the Secondary Use of Electronic Health Record Data," *EGEMs Gener. Evid. Methods Improve Patient Outcomes*, vol. 4, no. 1, p. 18, Sep. 2016, doi: 10.13063/2327-9214.1244.

[3]   C. O. Schmidt *et al.*, "Facilitating harmonized data quality assessments. A data quality framework for observational health research data collections with software implementations in R," *BMC Med. Res. Methodol.*, vol. 21, no. 1, p. 63, Dec. 2021, doi: 10.1186/s12874-021-01252-7.

[4]   M. Kiehntopf and K. W. Böer, *Biomaterialbanken: Checkliste zur Qualitätssicherung*. Berlin: Medizinisch-Wissenschaftliche Verl.-Ges, 2008.

---

4 https://dzhk.de/en/dzhk-heart-bank/submitting-applications/

5 Project Repository: https://gitlab.gwdg.de/medinfpub/data-quality-workflow

[5]   M. R. La Frano *et al.*, "Impact of post-collection freezing delay on the reliability of serum metabolomics in samples reflecting the California mid-term pregnancy biobank," *Metabolomics*, vol. 14, no. 11, p. 151, Nov. 2018, doi: 10.1007/s11306-018-1450-9.

[6]   L. M. Spekhorst *et al.*, "Cohort profile: design and first results of the Dutch IBD Biobank: a prospective, nationwide biobank of patients with inflammatory bowel disease," *BMJ Open*, vol. 7, no. 11, p. e016695, Nov. 2017, doi: 10.1136/bmjopen-2017-016695.

[7]   C.-J. L. Farrell and A. C. Carter, "Serum indices: managing assay interference," *Ann. Clin. Biochem. Int. J. Lab. Med.*, vol. 53, no. 5, pp. 527–538, Sep. 2016, doi: 10.1177/0004563216643557.

[8]   M. Cornes *et al.*, "European survey on preanalytical sample handling – Part 2: Practices of European laboratories on monitoring and processing haemolytic, icteric and lipemic samples. On behalf of the European Federation of Clinical Chemistry and Laboratory Medicine (EF," *Biochem. Medica*, vol. 29, no. 2, pp. 334–345, Jun. 2019, doi: 10.11613/BM.2019.020705.

[9]   T. Schwaneberg *et al.*, "Data privacy management and data quality monitoring in the German Centre for Cardiovascular Research's multicentre TranslatiOnal Registry for CardiomyopatHies (DZHK-TORCH): TORCH data quality management and monitoring," *ESC Heart Fail.*, vol. 4, no. 4, pp. 440–447, Nov. 2017, doi: 10.1002/ehf2.12168.

[10]   S. Herzinger *et al.*, "SmartR: an open-source platform for interactive visual analytics for translational research data," *Bioinformatics*, vol. 33, no. 14, pp. 2229–2231, Jul. 2017, doi: 10.1093/bioinformatics/btx137.

[11]   H. Spengler, I. Gatz, F. Kohlmayer, K. A. Kuhn, and F. Prasser, "Improving Data Quality in Medical Research: A Monitoring Architecture for Clinical and Translational Data Warehouses," in *2020 IEEE 33rd International Symposium on Computer-Based Medical Systems (CBMS)*, Rochester, MN, USA, Jul. 2020, pp. 415–420. doi: 10.1109/CBMS49503.2020.00085.

[12]   C. Blacketer, F. J. Defalco, P. B. Ryan, and P. R. Rijnbeek, "Increasing Trust in Real-World Evidence Through Evaluation of Observational Data Quality," Health Informatics, preprint, Mar. 2021. doi: 10.1101/2021.03.25.21254341.

German Medical Data Sciences 2022 - Future Medicine
R. Röhrig et al. (Eds.)
© *2022 The authors and IOS Press.*
This article is published online with Open Access by IOS Press and distributed under the terms
of the Creative Commons Attribution Non-Commercial License 4.0 (CC BY-NC 4.0).

Subject Index

German Medical Data Sciences 2022 - Future Medicine
R. Röhrig et al. (Eds.)

109

Author Index